T0277055

IMPERFECT CONCEPTIONS

FRANK DIKÖTTER

Imperfect Conceptions

Medical Knowledge, Birth Defects and Eugenics in China

COLUMBIA UNIVERSITY PRESS
NEW YORK

Columbia University Press
New York

Library of Congress Cataloging-in-Publication Data

Dikötter, Frank,
    Imperfect conceptions, medical knowledge, birth defects, and
eugenics in China/Frank Dikötter.
        p.   cm.
    Includes bibliographical references and index.
    ISBN 978-0-231-11370-0
    1. Abnormalities. Human–China–Public opinion. 2. Abnormalities,
Human–Etiology–Public opinion. 3. Eugenics–China. 4. Public
opinion–China. I. Title.
    RG627.2.C5D54 1998
    616', 043' 0951–dc21
                                                    98-15584
                                                       CIP

ACKNOWLEDGEMENTS

I acknowledge with gratitude the Research Fellowship of the Wellcome Trust for the History of Medicine which allowed me to carry out most of the research for this book, which was completed under a Wellcome University Award. A number of people have kindly shared their ideas and suggestions with me or read and commented on draft versions, in particular Dagmar Borchard, Berlin Free University; Delia Davin, University of Leeds; Harriet Evans, University of Westminster; Hsiung Ping-chen, Academia Sinica, Taipei; Terence H. Hull, Australian National University; Dorothy Ko, Rutgers University; Lars Laamann, University of Westminster; Martin Lau, SOAS; David Parkin, Oxford University; Veronica Pearson, University of Hong Kong; Stirling D. Scruggs, United Nations Population Fund, New York; Xun Zhou, SOAS; Nicolas Zufferey, University of Geneva. All errors and omissions are mine alone.

London, December 1997   F. D.

CONTENTS

ILLUSTRATIONS

'Sow melons and you will reap melons, plant beans and you will harvest beans.'   *Popular Saying*

'Superior intelligence and inferior stupidity cannot be changed.'   *The Analects*

1

INTRODUCTION

The People's Republic of China passed a law in 1995 aimed at restricting births deemed to be imperfect. It supports the systematic 'implementation of premarital medical check-ups' in order to detect whether one of the intending parents suffers from a 'serious hereditary', venereal or reproductive disorder as well as a 'relevant mental disorder' or 'legal contagious disease': it suggests that in order to prevent 'inferior births', those 'deemed unsuitable for reproduction' should undergo sterilisation or abortion or be compelled to remain celibate.[1]

This book looks at the broader historical, cultural, social and political context of eugenics in China. It claims that the 1995 law should be seen as part of a much wider eugenic campaign based on the dissemination of medical knowledge on reproductive health to the general public. A coercive vision which wishes to prevent the dissemination of 'unfit' people is combined with a more pedagogical approach, which seeks to impart a sense of reproductive responsibility to every individual. In the name of a more eugenic future, conjugal couples are enjoined strictly to monitor their reproductive behaviour and exercise self-discipline before, during and after conception. The choice of a partner, the age of marriage, the timing of conception and even the quality of the semen are all claimed to influence the health of future offspring significantly. The medical knowledge dispensed in eugenic campaigns is not designed to enable informed individual choices in reproductive matters, but to instil a moral message of sexual restraint and reproductive

---

1 'Zhonghua renmin gongheguo muying baojian fa' (The People's Republic of China's maternal and infant health law), *Zhonghua renmin gongheguo quanguo renmin daibiao dahui changwu weiyuanhui gongbao*, 1994, no. 7, pp. 3–8.

duty in the name of collective health. Eugenics promotes a biologising vision of society in which the reproductive rights of individuals are subordinated to the rights of an abstract collectivity.

It would be wrong to describe eugenics in the PRC as a marginal field dominated only by a few medical experts: it provides an over-arching rationale to very different concerns about reproductive health and social reform. Many important issues which are not related to eugenics in developed countries – such as the strains on local resources and families inseparable from maintaining individuals with disabilities, the desire to improve pre-natal screening techniques to achieve better levels of child health, and the need to provide genetic counselling for prospective parents – are articulated within and constrained by a policy which gives priority to the needs of the collectivity over the rights and choices of individuals. While some medical circles and government officials make laudable efforts to improve reproductive health, provide medical information and strengthen support systems for disabled individuals and have legitimate interests in achieving these aims, the motivation of many of them is embedded in a more general approach aimed at improving the 'quality' of the population. Eugenic concerns provide a coherent link and underlying rationale to such widespread issues as environmental pollution, reproductive technologies, population increase, migration patterns and even dietary habits: numerous aspects of modernity are related to a vision of national 'fitness'. Moreover, as in Scandinavian countries till the 1960s and '70s, many of these concerns are shared by important sections of the educated public.[2] In apparent refutation of the commonly accepted observation that eugenics declined rapidly in Europe after the Second World War, tens of thousands of people continued to be

2 Gunnar Broberg and Nils Roll-Hansen (eds), *Eugenics and the welfare state: Sterilization policy in Denmark, Sweden, Norway, and Finland*, East Lansing: Michigan State University Press, 1996.

sterilised in Finland, Denmark, Norway and Sweden up till 1960. Sterilisation laws were based on a large consensus among the population, since eugenics was seen as integral to a comprehensive programme of social reform in a developing welfare state. Concern about the number of mentally retarded people also contributed to some sort of consensus across the political spectrum on the necessity for mild eugenic measures. A far cry from the atrocities committed in Nazi Germany, eugenics in the PRC would be closer to the eugenics movement in the welfare states of Scandinavia. As in Europe up till the advent of a more open and affluent society in the 1960s, few voices in the PRC today question the scientific credibility and political implications of eugenic practices.

As is apparent from the example of Scandinavia, attempts to regulate the reproduction of individuals in the name of eugenics are not unique to the PRC. This book contends that recent developments in reproductive health in China are directly indebted to a eugenic vision elaborated between the two World Wars. The second part shows that eugenic discourse was already widespread in republican China, a period of drastic political, social and cultural change during which ideas of racial hygiene permeated almost every field related to human reproduction, from birth control to sex education. Eugenics was a fundamental aspect of some of the most important cultural and social movements of the twentieth century, intimately linked to ideologies of 'race', nation and sex. It was also part of a more global movement. As mounting evidence provided by historians of medicine shows, race improvement was far from being a politically conservative and scientifically spurious set of beliefs which remained confined to the Nazi era; it belonged on the contrary to the political vocabulary of almost every significant modernising force between the two World Wars. Till recently, the historiographical focus on the most extreme expressions of race improvement in Germany, Britain and the United States tended to perpetuate a one-sided representation which ignored the multifarious dimensions and extraordinary appeal of eugenics to individuals of very different social backgrounds, political convictions and nationalities. In China as in France, eugenics was part of such widely discussed themes as evolution, degeneration, civilisation and modernity, and touched on a wide variety of emerging fields like maternity, psychiatry, criminology, public health and sex education. It was supported by scientific societies, pressure groups and political institutions in countries as different as India, Brazil and Sweden. Widely seen as a morally acceptable and scientifically viable way of improving human heredity, it was embraced by social reformers, established intellectuals and medical authorities from one extreme of the political spectrum to the other, from British conservatives to Spanish anarchists.[3] Eugenics was not so much a clear set of scientific principles as a modern way of talking about social problems in biologising terms: politicians with mutually incompatible beliefs and scientists with opposed interests could all selectively appropriate eugenics to portray society as an organic body to be guided by biological laws. Eugenics gave scientific authority to social fears and moral panics, lent respectability to racial prejudice and class bias, and legitimised sterilisation acts and immigration laws. Powered by the prestige of science, eugenics allowed modernising élites to represent their prescriptive claims about social order as objective statements irrevocably grounded in the laws of nature.

3 The reference to Spain is from Richard Cleminson, 'Eugenics by name or nature? The Spanish anarchist sex reform of the 1930s', History of European Ideas, 18 (1994), pp. 729–40; some recent review articles provide useful overviews of the field, namely Frank Dikötter, 'Race culture: Recent perspectives on the history of eugenics', American Historical Review, 103, no. 2 (April 1998), pp. 467–78; Robert Nye, 'The rise and fall of the eugenics empire: Recent perspectives on the impact of bio-medical thought in modern society', Historical Journal, 36, no. 3 (1993), pp. 687–700; P. J. Pauly, 'Review article: The eugenics industry – Growth or restructuring?', Journal of the History of Biology, 26, no. 1 (spring 1993), pp. 131–45.

Eugenic discourse had different meanings to different social groups in different contexts: it was appropriated and used in a variety of ways to accommodate radically divergent purposes and interests, being flexible enough to unite individuals or constituencies with contradictory agendas. One of the major dividing lines within eugenic discourse was that between a hard approach to heredity, based on genetics in Britain and Germany, and a soft approach combining an emphasis on the environment with hereditarian explanations. The soft approach to eugenics was common in republican China as well as in other countries as diverse as Brazil and France. French medical experts, for instance, campaigned for better public education in social hygiene and sexual health in the name of race improvement. To some extent, medical experts in republican China would have agreed with the concluding statement made by the Latin Eugenic Congress in 1937, which was explicitly critical of the more interventionist ideas of Anglo-Saxon and German eugenists: 'Faith in educational action constitutes, in our opinion, the most appropriate way of ensuring that eugenics, as a discipline, achieves the superior ends it envisages, namely stopping the degeneration of individuals, nations and races and helping the[ir] continuous improvement. [...] The eugenic problem is first of all a pedagogical problem.'[4] Independently of his French and Italian contemporaries, Wang Chengpin exclaimed in 1939: 'To strengthen the country, one first has to strengthen the race; to strengthen the race, one first has to improve sex education.'[5]

Unlike researchers in countries which pursued a hard Mendelian approach, proponents of eugenics in China did not produce significant biological research or statistical stud-

4 Anne Carol, *Histoire de l'eugénisme en France. Les médecins et la procréation, XIXe–XXe siècle*, Paris: Seuil, 1995, p. 286.
5 Wang Chengpin, *Qingchun de xingjiaoyu* (Sex education for youth), Shanghai: Xiongdi chubanshe, 1939, p. 1.

ies. As in many other countries, notably France, race hygiene was part of the vocabulary of most political groups, from the far left to the extreme right, as many intellectuals shared a concern over modernity, a sense of nationalism and expectation that the government should reform society. An emphasis on the virtues of education accounts for the relative absence in republican China of formal institutions, official organs or professional organisations centred around the promotion of eugenic ideals. Rather than emanating from a solid organisational foundation, eugenic discourse was supported by a variety of voices in the social field: it attracted popular journalists, social reformers, medical writers, sex educators, university professors and political ideologues, all attempting to promote medical knowledge and reproductive health for the sake of a more eugenic nation. An exclusive focus on institutions or a narrow emphasis on legislative processes, in that sense, would fail to highlight the dispersed but prevalent nature of eugenic discourse in medical circles, political élites and professional groups in republican China. A shift away from prominent intellectuals towards the more anonymous supporters of eugenics, a greater focus on the reception of eugenics at more popular levels of culture, and a more sustained analysis of traditional hereditarian attitudes – these elements help to explain the widespread support for eugenic discourse between the two World Wars. Looking beyond the institutional boundaries of formal organisations, we find that eugenic discourse permeated the concerns of many ordinary men and women. As eugenics was popularised, it gave scientific credibility and respectability to attitudes, anxieties and values which were prevalent primarily if not exclusively among the formally educated levels of society.

Comparative approaches to the history of eugenics have highlighted the extent to which common medical knowledge has been mobilised and transformed by very distinct local styles of expression dependent on the political, economic, social and cultural variables of particular institutions, social groups or countries.[6] However, the importance of traditional ideas in the emergence of eugenics within specific cultures is rarely studied in any detail, although a few authors observe how popular hereditarian notions – encapsulated in such sayings as 'Like begets like' – strongly helped the emergence and acceptance of eugenic ideas. In France, for instance, eugenics was not simply a transplant from Britain, where Francis Galton and Karl Pearson had first heralded the 'science of race improvement'; well before 1860, French doctors envisaged the regulation of reproduction in order to improve the human race. The hereditary transmission of deleterious features, the need for matrimonial legislation, the physical degeneration of the human race and the medical administration of human reproduction are some of the ideas broached by medical authorities concerned by the progress of civilisation and the physical qualities of the population. In 1803 Louis Robert even proposed a new science called 'megalanthropologenesy': this would enable the government to identify men of superior abilities, select women of outstanding breeding talents, and closely monitor the entire reproductive process from insemination to delivery in state institutions. Traditional ideas associated with reproductive health, from the quality of sperm to the choice of a mating partner, also reappeared in the guise of eugenic science after 1860. Anne Carol sees elements of continuity running through medical ideas in France from the late eighteenth century to the present day, specifically emphasising soft inheritance, racial regeneration and reproductive health.[7]

Very similar ideas also circulated in China before the end of the nineteenth century, as the first part of this book demonstrates: many medical publications in late imperial China discussed in great detail ways of improving the physi-

6 Mark B. Adams (ed.), *The wellborn science: Eugenics in Germany, France, Brazil and Russia*, Oxford University Press, 1990.
7 Carol, *Histoire de l'eugénisme en France*.

cal quality of a line of descent while also highlighting the
medical dangers to future offspring of careless reproduction.
These older medical ideas contributed to the shaping of
eugenic discourse in the twentieth century: recasting more
traditional notions of reproductive health in the radically
new language of science, eugenic discourse in twentieth-
century China was more of a cultural reconfiguration structured by older modes of representation than a radical
rupture with 'tradition'. Just as traditional hereditarian attitudes and gender assumptions shaped eugenic discourse in
many European countries, eugenic ideas in China thrived
on patrilineal culture. Patrilineal culture, in which reproduction was represented as something potentially dangerous
that should be carefully regulated in order to safeguard the
lineage's future, permeated many medical publications in
the late imperial period. Individuals were represented as a
key element in a patrilineal line of descent, envisaged as an
indispensable link connecting past ancestors and future
descendants, and as such were enjoined to regulate and
administer their reproductive behaviour for the sake of the
lineage. The individual, seen in relationship to the lineage,
was held to be responsible not only for his or her own
reproductive behaviour, but also for the health of future offspring.

Medical approaches to reproductive health in the three historical periods considered here were also characterised by a
pervasive concern with birth defects. As in other countries
marked by gender inequalities, women were generally held
accountable for the appearance of babies judged to be malformed at birth. Imperfect conceptions, in a society in
which the status of a family has often been defined largely
by its ability to engender healthy offspring, were frequently
seen within the educated strata of society as undesirable.
Births of hermaphrodites, conjoined twins and other human

oddities were considered extraordinary events which merit-
ed detailed recording in the annals and, before the fall of the
empire in 1911, a full report to the Board of Rites.[8] More
generally, however, babies with severe physical disabilities
probably did not grow to adulthood in late imperial China,
although historical evidence to substantiate this hypothesis is
lacking. If medical discourse can be analysed by a cultural
historian to highlight how boundaries of normality and
abnormality were socially constructed in given periods,
most other written sources reveal little about the social
experiences of disabled people. In a patrilineal society
whose cultural preference for healthy sons was so strong that
even the birth of a girl was not mentioned in most genealogies, they left virtually no trace in the written record of
imperial China, except in a fictional guise in literary sketches on the strange (biji).[9] Where children with major disabilities were allowed to survive and grow up, their voices still
remain to be discovered. If the scarcity of significant primary sources makes a social history of the lives of individuals
deemed 'imperfect' all but impossible, a cultural historian
can examine the meanings with which births defects have
been endowed and investigate the broader cultural values
and social attitudes related to human reproduction.

Fascination with the deviant, the horror of otherness, the
desire to demarcate the normal from the abnormal are some
of the more important aspects that a cultural history of birth
defects would highlight. While a continuum of disabilities
appeared in medical texts, ranging from extreme cases of
malformation to mild defects, a focus on imperfect births
may also reveal more widespread notions of the human
body. For instance, in a holistic approach that denies the

8 Berthold Laufer, 'Sex transformation and hermaphrodites in China', *American
Journal of Physical Anthropology*, 3, no. 2 (1920), reprinted in *Kleinere Schriften von
Berthold Laufer*, Wiesbaden: Franz Steiner Verlag, 1979, part 2, pp. 1306–9.
9 See for instance Judith Zeitlin, *Historian of the strange: Pu Songling and his
Chinese classical tale*, Stanford University Press, 1993.

existence of a disembodied and autonomous self, medical discourse has closely related the individual to the environment. Hostile forces in the environment can cause illness in pregnant women and induce a variety of foetal disorders. Furthermore, causal power is attributed to pathogenic agents: whether spirits and demons in the late imperial period, or germs, microbes and toxins in the new medical vocabularies of the twentieth century, an ontological conception of disease in which pathological agents were seen to attack the pregnant woman stressed how insubstantial was the boundary between the human body and its social environment. However, malformations are never considered simply as the result of an unwholesome environment: a holistic approach also reinforces the link between social disorder and biological retribution. In the same way as, during the Qing, the sexually deviant thoughts of a woman were claimed to cause a ghost or spirit to take possession of her womb, the corrupt products of modernity are now held responsible for the chemicals and toxins that lead to birth defects. Simultaneous statements are thus made about the spiritual alienation of the modern individual and the biological estrangement of that individual's offspring. These examples point to the central role attributed to human responsibility in the aetiology of health in China: the illness of offspring is often analogically related to the moral failure of the progenitors. Minimising the relevance of less deterministic modes of interpretation, such as the randomness of genetic mutations or the unpredictability of embryological malformations, medical determinism is part of a mode of explanation of the universe in anthropocentric terms whereby human responsibility and personal behaviour appear fundamental. The analogies constructed between morality and health, the fear of excess and the importance of self-control are rearticulated in a medical discourse which represents the monster as biological retribution for social deviation. In this highly determined universe, birth defects are seen as a human failure which should be eliminated.

Medical holism emphasises the complementarity of body and mind and the interdependence between the human person and the environment. A holistic approach to human health should be distinguished from a holistic emphasis on group rights in which the individual is portrayed as a mere unit in a broader collectivity. Political holism, contrary to common belief, only became important in China with the advent of modernity. According to Ambrose King, the individual was seen in traditional China as a relational being, interacting with other concrete individuals in a network of personal role relations independent of any abstract group.[10] The relation between the individual and the group was ambiguous: the group, which had no definable boundaries and could be contracted or expanded at will, was given little theoretical emphasis in human ethics. Only with the emergence of a modern vision of the body politic was the individual explicitly related to a greater collectivity. Where few terms existed previously to envisage the relationship between individual and group, modernising intellectuals promoted a new political repertoire in an attempt to portray each person as an organic unit belonging to a larger collectivity, in terms of 'race' (*zhongzu*), 'population' (*renkou*), 'nation' (*minzu, guomin*), 'state' (*guojia*) and even 'gene pool' (*jiyinku*). We suggest that the emphasis on individual duties in the name of group rights is a thoroughly modern phenomenon which has little to do with 'traditional values'.

While this book highlights the significant social and political changes which took place from the late imperial period to the present, a detailed comparison between three different historical periods also questions the suggestion that 'modernity' inevitably entails a rupture with 'tradition' at all levels: as in the example of France, cited above, cultural reconfigurations rather than radical discontinuities are the

10 Ambrose Y.C. King, 'The individual and group in Confucianism' in Donald J. Munro, *Individualism and holism: Studies in Confucian and Taoist values*, Ann Arbor: Center for Chinese Studies, 1985, pp. 57–70.

characteristics of eugenic discourse in twentieth-century China. New ideas are understood through old ideas. As Marilyn Strathern has observed, advances in reproductive medicine often draw on ideas already in place, thus producing new forms out of old cultural material.[11] In a similar vein, patrilineal culture in China has both limited and made possible the choices offered by new medical knowledge. Consequently, this book explains eugenics in China not as a mere derivation of a more 'authentic' discourse from Europe, but as the result of an active process of appropriation located in a specific cultural, social and political context. Medical writers in China have understood eugenics in their own way, adapted science to their own use, and bent knowledge to their own needs. However, beyond these cultural specificities, eugenics in China is not significantly different from many movements for racial hygiene in Europe in its combination of a weak conception of individual rights with a strong biologising outlook: it proposes a politically conservative vision of the relationship between the state and the individual in the radically fashionable language of science. In other words, the identification of distinct approaches to and understandings of eugenics does not imply a recognition of their cultural relativity: one of the virtues of comparative history is to draw attention to the parochial and insular nature of many modernising discourses which use science as a legitimising force. That a one-party state in which the possibilities for the expression of dissenting voices is limited not only enables but actively promotes a vision of eugenic control only highlights the necessity for scholarly engagement.

---

11 Marilyn Strathern, *Reproducing the future: Anthropology, kinship and the new reproductive technologies*, Manchester University Press, 1992.

2

'IMPERFECT CONCEPTIONS': MEDICAL THEORIES AND BIRTH DEFECTS IN LATE IMPERIAL CHINA

INTRODUCTION

Medical theories on human conception circulated widely in late imperial China (*c.* 1550–1911). Well before the advent of medical science in the twentieth century, medical writers already advanced speculations about the nature of birth defects and proposed remedies which would promote the health of future offspring. Their interest in birth defects appeared in numerous books on women's health (*fuke*), childbirth (*chanke*) and paediatrics (*erke*), notably in chapters on 'seeking descendants' (*qiusi*) and 'planting a son' (*zhongzi*). Based on an analysis of about fifty such popular medical handbooks, this chapter shows that medical knowledge proposed many prohibitions, restrictions and injunctions on the behaviour of prospective parents in general and pregnant women in particular. Gestation was understood as a malleable process which could be positively influenced from the moment of conception to the point of delivery. The control of sexual desire, the timing of intercourse, the regulation of emotions, the supervision of a pregnant woman's diet were seen as important factors which could contribute to the health of the foetus. In a society structured around the lineage and its need for male descendants, the unborn child became the point of convergence of a number of very different interests, all thriving on the deployment of medical discourse: mothers wished to increase control over their own reproductive health, wealthy fathers sought to enlarge their families through the procreation of healthy sons, medical experts aspired to heighten their social status through the promotion of a body of specialised medical knowledge, conservative scholars attempted to assert their moral leadership through an emphasis on correct behaviour and proper discipline, and government officials were eager to protect the family and the lineage by insisting that sexual intercourse be confined to the household.

The source material on which this chapter is based belongs to the educated Confucian segment of the coastal region and is by no means representative of more popular approaches to health, as exemplified by mystic healers, itinerant medicine peddlers or rural midwives. Till well into the twentieth century, only the wealthy élites of important cities and towns patronised scholar-physicians, while large segments of the rural hinterland had recourse to village practitioners and healers who used a variety of therapeutic practices, from demonological medicine to religious healing in which altars were built to appease the spirits of disease. Within these alternative approaches to health and medicine, birth defects may have been seen in a different light, although the present state of the field does not allow the historian to substantiate such a hypothesis. For instance, popular deities could have weird bodily shapes and facial features, while even within Confucianism some of the mythical founders of ancient dynasties sometimes stood out by their strange physical appearance. Among ordinary people of the coastal region, however, new-born babies may not have been seen as having an intrinsic right to life, and poor farmers in the hinterland who could not even afford to keep a baby girl may have been ill-disposed towards any visible defects in infant boys. Compassionate families may have decided to keep, protect and care for a baby with a visible defect, although substantial evidence of any consistent medical or moral support for such individual attitudes has yet to be found.

Moreover, even within scholarly circles precious little was written about those liminal figures in society defined as physically or mentally abnormal. Contrary to the rich variety of source material in modern Europe,[1] ranging from scholarly case-studies of 'monsters' to widespread broadsheets on 'freak shows', the more formal and normative written traces left behind by the local élites in late imperial China say little about either the medical incidence of or the social attitudes towards people with deformities. An occasional sentence may surface here and there, revealing for instance that an eccentric scholar-official like Gong Zizhen had a head of unusual shape and was of small stature, but little is said about how this might have affected his personal life.[2] The biographies of scholar-officials can be fruitfully scanned to look at childhood diseases, but they do not in general comment on medical problems at birth.[3]

An unusual physical appearance was interpreted negatively in the art of physiognomy (*xiangshu or xiangfa*), namely the detection of inauspicious personal destinies in irregular

1 An important source of inspiration for the present study has been the work of Georges Canguilhem, in particular his 'La monstruosité et le monstrueux' in *La connaissance de la vie*, Paris: Vrin, 1992, pp. 171–84; a classic study is Jean Céard, *La nature et les prodiges*, Geneva: Droz, 1977; other useful studies include Albert Sonderegger, *Missgeburten und Wundergestalten in Einblattdrucken und Handzeichnungen des 16. Jahrhunderts*, Zürich: Füssli, 1927; Etienne Wolff, *La science des monstres*, Paris: Gallimard, 1948; Jean-Louis Fisher, *Monstres. Histoire du corps et de ses défauts*, Paris: Syros, 1992; K. Park and L.J. Daston, 'Unnatural conceptions: The study of monsters in sixteenth- and seventeenth-century France and England', *Past and Present*, no. 92 (August 1981), pp. 20–54; Patrick Tort, *L'ordre et les monstres. Le débat sur l'origine des déviations anatomiques au XVIIIe siècle*, Paris: Le Sycomore, 1980; M.T. Walton, R.M. Fineman and P. J. Walton, 'Of monsters and prodigies: The interpretation of birth defects in the sixteenth century', *American Journal of Medical Genetics*, 47, no. 1 (Aug. 1993), pp. 7–13; Dudley Wilson, *Signs and portents: Monstrous births from the Middle Ages to the Enlightenment*, London: Routledge, 1993.
2 Dorothy V. Borei, 'Eccentricity and dissent: The case of Kung Tzu-chen', *Ch'ing-shi wen-t'i*, 3, no. 4 (Dec. 1975), p. 51.
3 Hsiung Ping-chen, 'Zhongguo jinshi shiren bixia de ertong jiankang wenti' (Problems of child health in the writings of the educated élite in early modern China), *Zhongyang yanjiuyuan jindaishi yanjiusuo jikan*, 23, no. 2 (June 1994), pp. 1–29.

facial features. Popular encyclopaedias like the *Sancai tuhua*, for instance, included detailed lists of inauspicious facial features,[4] while the *Santai wanyong zhengzong* went so far as to identify 'thieves' and 'paupers' on the basis of physical appearance.[5] More generally, the incidence of deaf, blind, mute, hunchbacked or otherwise disabled children must have been fairly high in any society before the advent of systematic child and maternal health care. A discursive silence may be reflective of a social liminality to which children with birth defects are still reduced in many countries today, including the People's Republic of China: their low visibility in the cities and towns of the coastal regions is in itself an indication of social prejudice, as if those defined as abnormal are allowed to live only within the confines of their families, taking care not to offend society by appearing in public. The limited nature of the available sources, rather than any particular ideological reason, thus directs a preliminary inquiry into a cultural and social history of birth defects towards an analysis of medical discourse among the small élite of scholar-physicians in the late imperial period.

ÉLITE MEDICAL THEORIES IN LATE IMPERIAL CHINA

A medical focus on sexual intercourse and reproductive health appeared well before the end of the Ming. Traditional sex handbooks, which circulated among the élites from the Han (206 BC – AD 220) to the Tang (618–907) dynasties, already closely integrated sexual practices with personal health and generative strength. The 'art of the bedchamber' (*fangzhong*) favoured sexual techniques for 'returning semen' (*huanjing*) in order to promote conju-

4 Wang Qi and Wang Siyi, *Sancai tuhua* (Illustrated encyclopaedia), repr. Shanghai: Shanghai guji chubanshe, 1988, vol. 2, pp. 1474–91.
5 Yu Xiangdou, *Santai wanyong zhengzong* (Encyclopaedia), orig. 1599, *juan* 30. This reference was given to me by Dorothy Ko.

gal harmony, personal longevity and reproductive health. The preservation of bodily fluids such as semen, saliva and vaginal secretions was seen as a means of increasing one's primordial vitality and harnessing cosmic energies that presided over life and death.[6] Moreover, after the seventh century medical writers increasingly shifted their emphasis away from male bodies to emphasise women as the primary agent of reproduction, offering medical recipes for women and advice on maternal health care. Reproductive medicine proposed techniques to enhance conception and protect the foetus in order to engender a healthy son.[7]

The earlier 'art of the bedchamber' lost some of its sway after the rise of Cheng-Zhu Confucianism under the Southern Song (1127–1279): advocating a strict adherence to Confucian principles after the Jurchens swept over the north of the country, Cheng-Zhu scholarship rapidly gained acceptance, and by 1240 had become state orthodoxy.[8] Disciplined self-cultivation and introspection, a commitment to moral transformation and orthodox education: Cheng-Zhu scholars emphasised 'the preservation of heavenly principles and the elimination of human desires' (cun tianli mie renyu). Traditional books exclusively dedicated to sexual techniques were marginalised under the political and ideological orthodoxy of Cheng-Zhu Confucianism. 'Human desires', put forward in opposition to 'heavenly

---

6 Zhou Yimou, *Mawangdui Hanmu chutu: Fangzhong yangsheng* (The Mawangdui excavations from Han tombs: The art of the bedchamber and the nourishment of life), Hong Kong: Haifeng chubanshe, 1990; Douglas Wile, *Art of the bedchamber: The Chinese sexual yoga classics including women's solo meditation texts*, Albany: State University of New York Press, 1992; see also Robert Hans van Gulik, *Sexual life in ancient China*, Leiden: E.J. Brill, 1974.

7 Li Jen-der, 'Han Tang zhijian qiuzi yifang shitan: jianlun fuke lanshang yu xingbie lunshu' (Reproductive medicine in late antiquity and early medieval China: Gender discourse and the birth of gynecology), *Zhongyang yanjiuyuan lishi yuyan yanjiu jikan*, 68, no. 2 (July 1997), pp. 283–367.

8 James T.C. Liu, *China turning inwards: Intellectual-political changes in the early twelfth century*, Cambridge, MA: Harvard University Press, 1988.

principles', were represented as potentially dangerous drives that should be eliminated for the sake of individual cultivation and social order, and sexual intercourse in particular was understood as a procreative act to be performed mainly in relation to marital fertility. Building on the seventh-century focus on female fertility, debates on human sexuality were confined to a few chapters on reproduction in medical treatises about women's health.

A number of important texts on medicine for women also appeared from the Song to the early Ming,[9] but health manuals only started to proliferate from the sixteenth century onwards. In the field of women's health, for instance, only three publications have been preserved from 1279 to 1548. More than a dozen treatises are known to have appeared in the century preceding the collapse of the Ming (1644), followed by well over 100 publications during the Qing (1644–1911).[10] A huge discursive inflation during the same period can also be found in other medical specialisations such as medicine for children (*erke*) and the 'nourishment of life' (*yangsheng*).[11] Of course, the mere appearance of a medical text is not in itself a viable indicator of its cul-

9 See Kong Shuzhen, 'Songdai fuchan kexue' (Medicine for childbirth and women in the Song dynasty), *Zhonghua yishi zazhi*, 1994, no. 3, pp. 183–5.

10 Xue Qinglu (ed.), *Quanguo zhongyi tushu lianhe mulu* (Combined catalogue of publications in Chinese medicine), Beijing: Zhongyi guji chubanshe, 1991, pp. 428–49.

11 On maternal and infant health care in late imperial China, see the work of Hsiung Ping-chen, *Youyou. Chuantong Zhongguo de qiangbao zhi dao* (The care of infants in traditional China), Taibei: Lianjing chuban shiye gongsi, 1995, as well as other titles by the author given below; see also Yi-Li Wu, 'Transmitted secrets: The doctors of the lower Yangzi region and "medicine for women" in late imperial China', Yale University, Ph.D. dissertation, 1998; for a list of useful references, see Ma Dazheng, *Zhongguo fuchanke fazhan shi* (History of medicine for women and childbirth in China), Taiyuan: Shanxi kexue jiaoyu chubanshe, 1991; on the extraordinary growth and dissemination of texts on health and longevity from the late Ming onwards, see Li Chunsheng, 'Ming Qing zhi jiefang qian yangsheng fazhan shi gai' (An overview of the history of the unfolding of *yangsheng* from the Ming and the Qing to liberation), *Zhonghua yishi zazhi*, 1989, 19, no. 2, pp. 71–5.

tural and social significance. The provincial and local histories of the late Ming and Qing, for instance, contain impressive lists of works on women's health and childbirth, as well as on smallpox and typhoid fever. Many of these publications were only of local significance and are no longer readily available, although their mere quantity indicates a remarkable dissemination of medical knowledge in late imperial China.[12] Some popular treatises, on the other hand, were frequently reprinted. The *Dashengbian* (Book on successful childbirth) of 1715, one of the most widely-circulated booklets on reproductive health,[13] was reprinted no less than eighty-four times before the fall of the empire in 1911. In contrast, Sun Simo's notorious *Beiji qianjin yaofang* (Essential prescriptions), first compiled in 652 and considered a medical classic, was only reprinted twice in the seventeenth century, while no other reprints appeared in China before 1849. The success of a given publication, in other words, was as much influenced by popular demand and commercial interest as by élite notions of textual value.

Commercial companies like the Xin'an printing house in Anhui province thrived on the publication of medical books, a trend indicative of the influence and importance of medical activities during the late Ming and the Qing.[14] Many of these books of vulgarisation, which reflect the common areas of interest between the reading public, medical experts and publishing houses, were printed with the financial assistance of local élites, often including rich mer-

12 Ho Ping-ti, *Studies on the population of China, 1368–1953*, Cambridge, MA: Harvard University Press, 1959, p. 327, n. 69.

13 See Jia Zhizhong and Yang Yanfei, '*Dashengbian* ji qi zuozhe kao' (An inquiry into the *Dashengbian* and its author), *Zhonghua yishi zazhi*, 1994, 24, no. 3, pp. 183–5.

14 Tong Guangdong, Wang Letao and Xu Yecheng, 'Ming Qing shiqi Hui ban yiji qi yishi zuoyong' (Medical publications printed in Anhui during the Ming and the Qing and their function in medical history), *Zhonghua yishi zazhi*, 1989, 19, no. 4, pp. 242–6.

20   MEDICAL THEORIES AND BIRTH DEFECTS

chants, as in Sichuan province.[15] In the Jiangnan region, the
successful Huanduzhai not only accommodated the perceived needs of readers, but also combined medical publishing and charity by distributing their publications cheaply or
free of charge. Some of their medical books were specifically
addressed to a broad audience. Such a one was an *Outline to
Women's Health*, which asserted that 'ordinary people will
keep a copy at their fingertips and display it as a great treasure of an orderly home'.[16] From the mid-sixteenth century
onwards, medical texts flooded the market, and many went
through reprints in different regions or were copied by
hand. Committed to making their medical publications
accessible to a general readership, local élites, medical writers and religious organisations often presented advice on
health in simple rhymes or question-and-answer manuals.
Punctuation marks, vocabulary aids and simple commentaries were offered in attempts to popularise more specialised fields of medical knowledge. Encyclopaedias and
cheap handbooks also made medical knowledge available to
a much larger section of the reading public, which also
included women.[17]

Distributed by a print culture which flourished as the
result of changing economic and social conditions as well as
higher rates of literacy,[18] medical publications which cen-

15 He Zhongjun, 'Wan Qing Sichuan puji leiyizhu de chansheng he yingxiang'
(The production and influence of medical books of vulgarisation in Sichuan
during the late Qing), *Zhonghua yishi zazhi*, 1994, 24, no. 1, pp. 20–2.
16 Ellen Widmer, 'The Huanduzhai of Hangzhou and Suzhou: A study in
seventeenth-century publishing', *Harvard Journal of Asiatic Studies*, 56, no. 1
(1996), pp. 117 and 101–2.
17 On women and commercial publishing in the seventeenth century, see
Dorothy Ko, *Teachers of the inner chambers: Women and culture in seventeenth-century
China*, Stanford University Press, 1994, pp. 29–67.
18 Evelyn S. Rawski, *Education and popular literacy in Ch'ing China*, Ann Arbor:
University of Michigan Press, 1979; Cynthia Brokaw, *The ledgers of merit and
demerit: Social change and moral order in late imperial China*, Princeton University
Press, 1991.

tred on fertility, longevity and reproductive health catered to a broad readership in the urban centres of the coastal region. At the same time, new forms of medical literature thrived on the expansion of semi-literate practitioners, female healers (regarded as unskilled), drug peddlers and charlatans, and these directly threatened the status of established medical experts of classical learning. The blurring of social distinctions by increased economic prosperity, the growth of a culture of conspicuous consumption, greater social mobility and a heightened competition over status all had an impact on the diffusion of medical specialisations throughout the late imperial period.[19]

The authority conferred by medical knowledge attracted a great diversity of writers, from the anonymous pamphlet on reproductive health compiled by a local savant to the learned treatise written by a distinguished scholar-official. Several factors combine to explain the popularity of medical knowledge. The ideal of state responsibility for the health of the population, established by the imperial sponsorship of medical education and assistance in the Song and Yuan dynasties, was increasingly eroded during the late Ming.[20] In response to the gradual decline of government intervention in medical matters, privately sponsored efforts at medical assistance by local notables, acting as philanthropists, developed under the Qing. By the 1560s, the great majority of charitable pharmacies and medical bureaux set up under the previous dynasties were no longer functioning. Growing

---

19 For an introduction, see Evelyn S. Rawski, 'Economic and social foundations of late imperial culture' in David Johnson, Andrew J. Nathan and Evelyn S. Rawski (eds), *Popular culture in late imperial China*, Berkeley: University of California Press, 1985, pp. 3–33; Linda Cooke Johnson (ed.), *Cities of Jiangnan in late imperial China*, Albany: State University of New York Press, 1993; Fan Shuzhi, *Ming Qing Jiangnan shizhen tanwei* (Studies on the cities of Jiangnan in the Ming and Qing), Shanghai: Fudan daxue chubanshe, 1990.
20 This section is largely based on Angela K. C. Leung, 'Organized medicine in Ming-Qing China: State and private medical institutions in the Lower Yangzi region', *Late Imperial China*, 8, no. 1 (June 1987), pp. 134–66.

involvement in medical aid and organised charity characterised the local élites of the Jiangnan region, particularly
with the wave of epidemics of the 1640s. Under the guid-
ance of these élites, local institutions like dispensaries and
infirmaries continued to develop in the Qing era, while
philanthropic activism was justified as an attempt to rectify
human failings in a retributive explanation which portrayed
epidemics as a punishment from Heaven for moral decay.

The decline in the availability of official positions, on
which the authority of the literati was ultimately based, also
contributed to a growing interest in medicine. Since the
number of vacant positions for government officials remained
constant despite very rapid population growth, many scholars
were forced to pursue alternative careers, either as 'men of
culture' (wenren), a life-style increasingly popular in the
Ming and the Qing, or as more specialised experts capable
of offering pragmatic knowledge.

Redefinitions of scholarship brought about an emphasis
on more precise fields of knowledge or on the acquisition
of alternative skills, and a growing number of scholars
turned their attention towards medicine. Cultural reorienta-
tions – in particular a shift from philosophical speculation to
practical learning, the critical examination of classical texts
and the rise of evidential scholarship – further created an
environment conducive to the expansion of medical knowledge. After the fall of the Ming, the widespread compilation
of encyclopaedias, initiated by the Qing in order to rally
support from scholars, also furthered the circulation of
medical knowledge. One example is the influential Golden
Mirror of Medicine (Yizong jinjian), compiled by Wu Qian, a
member of the Imperial Academy of Medicine in the second half of the eighteenth century. In an endeavour to
propagate preventive medicine, the Golden Mirror carried
important sections on maternal and infant health care which
presented contemporary knowledge in simple prose or
rhymed verses.

Although increased competition over different fields of

knowledge led to an expansion in the number of medical specialists who sought to sell their advice on reproductive problems, medical knowledge on human reproduction underwent no major transformations in late imperial China comparable to those in Europe. In a highly mobile society centred around the maintenance of social status, scholars tended to identify and affiliate more closely with groups and schools of thought rather than asserting their own individuality in the pursuit of new knowledge. Essays and commentaries, the most important means of exchanging knowledge among scholars in imperial China, were often less concerned with the discovery of new factual evidence and the display of individual achievements in research than with the drawing of demarcation lines between different strands of thought and the identification of genealogies of knowledge to which the author could claim allegiance.

Two major schools in particular appear to have contributed to the development of reproductive theories. Many writers invoked the scholarship of Zhu Zhenheng (Danxi, 1281–1358), one of the key medical practitioners of the Yuan dynasty influenced by Zhu Xi and Zhou Dunyi. In their emphasis on the virtues of quiescence (*jing*), followers of the Danxi school claimed that *yin* was always deficient and *yang* always in excess. The 'monarchical' fire (*junhuo*) and 'minesterial' fire (*xianghuo*) – some medical terms were based on an analogy between the human body and the body politic – respectively located in the liver and the kidney (seen as a single viscera which stored the essence of life), consumed *yin* energy which could become depleted and should be nourished by medication. The Danxi school also insisted on the regulation of desire (*jieyu*), because indulgence in sexual intercourse would inflame the kidney and waste semen. Blood and semen both belonged to *yin* and could easily be dissipated. Cooling medications (*lianghan*) were often prescribed, including herbs to replenish the kidney like rhizome of rehmanniam (*shengdihuang*) and the bark of the Chinese corktree (*huangbo*). Dai Sigong (1323–1405), an important follower of Zhu Zhenheng, treated a number of illnesses on this basis: nocturnal emissions, for instance, were thought to be caused by excessive heat which could stimulate the storage of semen.

The Danxi school was mainly located in southern Jiangsu and northern Zhejiang, and competed with the Dongyuan school, allegedly founded by Li Mingzhi (Li Gao) and influential in Hebei (Zhongzhou). Other voices were raised against Zhu Zhenheng – for example, the followers of Xue Ji (ca. 1488–1558), who on the contrary emphasised the need to 'warm up and replenish' (wenbu). An influential author of many medical works, he supported the principle that the spleen and the kidney should be replenished with medications. Followers of the Dongyuan school, in particular Wan Quan and Wang Kentang, also insisted on the replenishment of the spleen and stomach and strongly opposed cooling medications. A third trend combined some elements of the Danxi and Dongyuan schools in considering the 'gate of life' (mingmen) to be the main regulator of the human body: the strength or weakness of its fire determined a person's vitality. Zhang Jiebin and Zhao Xianke's theory which stressed the 'nourishment of the yin, warming and replenishment' (ziyin wenbu) to increase vitality was also popular.

Despite different individual and regional approaches to medical prescriptions, however, there was a great amount of overlap in health manuals in the late Ming and Qing, since they invoked similar theories, drew on the same authors, quoted from identical texts and generally adopted a relatively uniform outlook. Whatever the approach of these different authors, from the late Ming onwards medical prescriptions were hugely popular products. The Xin'an dispensaries in Anhui province, which were closely linked to the printing house of the same name mentioned above, grew during the Ming to reach a peak under the Qing. They were mainly run by physicians up till the fall of the

Ming, after which they were taken over by merchants from Anhui.[21] Even distinguished authors sometimes linked their written work to a thriving business in medical products; one such was Wang Ji (Wang Shishan, 1463–1539), a famous sixteenth-century medical expert who opened a store in Qimen.[22]

If different authors invoked a variety of approaches to medication, all emphasised the importance of control to the maintenance of health: physical strength and generative power were thought to be determined at least in part by a person's life-style and not by fate or destiny alone. In its conception of the person, medical discourse focused more on the inner mechanisms of human bodies than on cosmological forces. These medical publications, moreover, discussed sex almost exclusively in terms of human reproduction; medical discourse drew on the pathological consequences of sexual excess for the health of future progeny. Vital energy seemed to be located inside the body itself, centred on the reproductive organs, and could be enhanced by a disciplined approach to sexual intercourse. Many medical publications contained long lists of prescriptions, since vitality and longevity were believed to be enhanced by the use of medications.

As followers of the Dongyuan and Danxi schools increasingly criticised ancient recipes contained in the classics of medicine, alternative recipes flourished, particularly in the sixteenth and seventeenth centuries. Confusion soon spread, as the contemporary Wang Lun complained: 'Books of the schools of Dongyuan and Danxi circulate widely in our society, and today's doctors, noticing that their prescriptions

21 Tong Guangdong and Liu Huiling, 'Ming Qing shiqi Xin'an yaodian ji qi yiyaoxue zuoyong' (Xin'an dispensaries and their role in the Ming and Qing), *Zhonghua yishi zazhi*, 1995, 25, no. 1 , pp. 30–4.
22 See Sheng Weizhong, '*Waike lili* ji Wang Ji de waike xueshu sixiang' (The *Principles of Surgery* of Wang Ji and his knowledge of surgery), *Zhonghua yishi zazhi*, 1985, 15, no. 1 , pp. 48–53.

are not the same as those of the ancients, all blindly imitate them; with the proliferation of prescriptions, the nature of the drugs is unclear, many are prescribed in an indiscriminate and hurried way and have no effect, adversely affecting the illness, so it becomes difficult to cure.'[23] Huang Yuanyu, a medical writer who lost an eye as the consequence of incorrect treatment, was also virulent in his denunciation of the Dongyuan and Danxi schools. Although he used *wenbu* prescriptions, he was scathing about Xue Ji, Zhang Jiebin, Zhao Xianke and others who used ingredients that are not mentioned in the classics, and was particularly critical of medications to replenish the yin (*ziyin*). Like other seventeenth- and eighteenth-century Han Confucianists, who attacked the medical schools which had flourished after the Song and promoted a return to a strict interpretation of the classics, Xu Dachun (1693–1771) discouraged the use of tonics and only recommended consumption of the five grains after an illness. Similar ideas appeared in the comments on medical classics by other scholars of classical learning like Yu Chang and You Yi. Many of these debates were related to the consolidation of patrilineal culture under the Qing, to be discussed in the next section.

MEDICAL DISCOURSE AND THE CONSOLIDATION OF THE LINEAGE UNDER THE QING

None of the core elements of medical knowledge in late imperial China was entirely original, since many were rearticulated, reconfigured or simply given a new emphasis in an approach which stressed the responsibility of the individual in engendering healthy offspring. Concern over the health of future progeny may also have been influenced by demographic changes. Ho Ping-ti has asserted that the division of family, the dilution of wealth due to the absence of

---

23 Fan Xingzhun, *Zhongguo yixue shilüe* (Essentials of history of Chinese medicine), Beijing: Zhongyi guji chubanshe, 1986, p. 202.

primogeniture and the pressures of downward mobility led to a greater emphasis on family instructions, austere puritanism and the values of self-discipline. Conspicuous consumption in order to maintain social status caused a dilution of wealth and consequent downward mobility, a trend that was sometimes accompanied by the failure of some families to reproduce themselves biologically. Ho speculates that this might have been due to an excess of sensual pleasures and other forms of dissipation.[24] Social anxiety over healthy reproduction, and in particular the fear of a decline in fertility together with a loss of social status, may have contributed to the huge interest in medical books in late imperial China.[25] A serial analysis of life-spans on the basis of lineage genealogies might provide evidence for a correlation between fertility and wealth,[26] but is clearly beyond the scope of this chapter.

Genealogical books generally did not record any information about births of children with malformations; as in most societies before the end of the nineteenth century, few probably survived to adulthood. Poor families may have been unable to care for babies with significant disabilities, and thus forced by sheer destitution to expose or abandon them. While charitable organisations were set up by local élites in the wealthier regions of China to combat infanticide, little has become known hitherto about the care for disabled infants in orphanages.[27] The incidence of disability,

24 Ho Ping-ti, *The ladder of success in imperial China: Aspects of social mobility, 1368–1911*, New York: Da Capo Press, 1976, pp. 138 and 162.

25 Of direct interest to these questions is Hsiung Ping-chen, 'More or less: Cultural and medical factors behind marital fertility in late imperial China', paper presented at the IUSSP/IRCJS Workshop, Kyoto, 17–22 Oct. 1994.

26 Stevan Harrell, 'The rich get children: Segmentation, stratification, and population in three Chekiang lineages, 1550–1850' in Susan B. Hanley and Arthur P. Wolf, *Family and population in East Asian history*, Stanford University Press, 1985, pp. 81–109.

27 See Angela K. C. Leung, *Shishan yu jiaohua: Ming Qing de cishan zuzhi* (Charity and civilisation: Charitable organisations in the Ming and the Qing), Taibei: Lianjing chuban shiye gongsi, 1997, pp. 85–95.

in any event, must have been fairly high in any society before the advent of systematic maternal and child health care in the twentieth century. For instance, the results of a historical investigation of a rural village in northern China reveal a high proportion of children born with various disabilities.[28] Poor maternal health may also have contributed to a high incidence of birth defects. Many mothers suffered from poor health and a weak constitution, to the point of being deficient in breast-milk – like the mother of Zuo Zongtang, a famous late Qing provincial leader.[29] The hardship of child-bearing was so great that many women sought medical intervention to avoid or end their pregnancies. The abuse of abortifacients in turn reinforced poor maternal health. The sixteenth-century scholar Gui Youguang (1506–71) was one among others who remembered how his mother lost her voice and later her overall health as the consequence of taking an abortifacient potion of snails. The difficulties that many mothers experienced only compounded the health problems of their children, who were easy prey to smallpox and other diseases. Poor maternal health and the medical complications induced by medications taken for contraceptive purposes no doubt also affected foetal health, and it could be hypothesised that the use of abortifacients might have enlarged the number of malformed babies.

On the other hand, significant developments in infant health care from at least the seventeenth century onwards probably had a positive impact on the survival rates of the

28 James Lee and Robert Eng, 'Population and family history in eighteenth-century Manchuria: Preliminary results from Daoyi, 1774–1798', *Ch'ing-shih wen-t'i*, 5, no. 1 (June 1984), pp. 1–55; see also James Z. Lee and Cameron D. Campbell, *Fate and fortune in rural China: Social organization and popular behaviour in Liaoning, 1774–1873*, Cambridge University Press, 1997.

29 The following two examples are taken from Hsiung Ping-chen, 'Constructed emotions: The bond between mothers and sons', *Late Imperial China*, 15, no. 1 (June 1994), p. 91; see also Hsiung Ping-chen, 'Sons and mothers: Demographic realities and the Chinese culture of *hsiao*', paper presented at the Annual Meeting of the Association of Asian Studies, Hawaii, 11–14 April 1996.

new-born.[30] As medical practices improved, including for instance wiping of the mouth, breaking the cord, bandaging the stump, washing the baby and expelling the new-born's faeces, medical practitioners also began looking for ways to save those at risk from difficult or premature birth or from birth defects. Efforts to care for the critically ill mainly took the form of a growing concern for maintaining the infant's body warmth and a search for various devices to rescue babies born in precarious conditions. From the late Ming onwards, some medical pamphlets began devoting chapters specifically to abnormal neonatal conditions, although most efforts were focused on healthy infants without physiological impediments. More generally, as this chapter shows, medical knowledge in the Ming and Qing increasingly included observations on birth defects and deformed babies, who were routinely referred to as 'incomplete in form' (*xingti buquan*) or 'deficient in form' (*xingti canji*). However, even within relatively wealthy circles medicine may not necessarily have played an exclusive role. Whether confronted with mild defects at birth or neonatal diseases, many families may have preferred to turn to religion and prayed to local gods, Buddhist figures or Daoist deities. The use of medications prepared within the household without outside help was also a widespread practice against which medical practitioners had to compete.[31]

Anxiety about healthy offspring was probably related to women's low social status in late imperial China. Women were often dependent on the production of healthy male offspring in order to improve their status in the family and in society. As Hsiung Ping-chen thoughtfully points out, in a gender hierarchy which inhibited the social mobility of women, the personal ambitions and social recognition to

30 See Hsiung Ping-chen, 'Zhongguo jinshi de xinsheng'er zhaohu' (Care for neonates in early modern China), *Zhongguo jinshi shehui wenhua shilun wenji* (Papers on society and culture in early modern China), Taibei: Academia Sinica, 1992, pp. 387–428.
31 Hsiung, 'Jinshi shiren', pp. 18–21.

which a woman aspired were best achieved by being the mother of a successful son.[32] Interest in the education and future career of a son was sometimes stronger in mothers than in fathers, since they often personally instructed their sons in the early years of formation, chose their lessons and selected instructional methods. Care in old age was literally dependent on the permanent allegiance, recognition and achievement of a son, not only within sections of the gentry but also among merchants and artisans. Popular ideas of foetal education (*taijiao*), which advanced the notion that the foetus could be educated *in utero*, played upon this need to secure a position in society through the success of one's offspring. If some medical writers were addressing a female readership, others specifically targeted illiterate women, and enjoined their husbands to read out the essentials of reproductive health in order to combat the nefarious influences on childbirth imputed to midwives.[33] Wang Yanchang went so far as to advocate regular readings of the popular *Dashengbian* (Book on successful childbirth) by the head of the family so that women would thoroughly master medical knowledge on human reproduction.[34]

The desire for healthy offspring was not confined to families. If fathers wished to display their social status through the production of healthy sons, and mothers sought to increase control over their own reproductive health, conservative scholars attempted to consolidate their moral leadership by emphasising correct behaviour and discipline.[35]

32 Hsiung, 'Constructed emotions', p. 97.
33 Xu Tingzhe, *Baochan yaozhi* (Essentials of childbirth), orig. 1806, 1898 edn, *juan* 1, p. 14b.
34 Wang Yanchang, *Wangshi yicun* (Medical writings of Wang Yanchang), orig. 1871, Hangzhou: Jiangsu kexue jishu chubanshe, 1983, pp. 129–30.
35 This section draws heavily on Kai-wing Chow, *The rise of Confucian ritualism in late imperial China: Ethics, Classics, and lineage discourse*, Stanford University Press, 1994; see also Kung-chuan Hsiao, *Rural China: Imperial control in the nineteenth century*, Seattle: University of Washington Press, 1967; Hilary J. Beattie, *Land and lineage in China: A study of T'ung-ch'eng County, Anhwei, in the Ming and Ch'ing dynasties*, Cambridge University Press, 1979.

After the conquest of China by the Manchus and the establishment of the Qing dynasty in 1644, the court provided the gentry with the stability and authority necessary to implement a conservative agenda of reform. Conservative sections of the gentry attempted to reclaim moral leadership and to reassert their duty to their local communities. The increased control over popular culture exercised by the Manchu court in the seventeenth century was supported by high officials and eminent scholars, in particular the followers of the Cheng-Zhu school of Confucianism. A return to the classics and a search for pure Confucianism also led to articulation of a deep concern over ritual practice. The strict observance of rites, in particular those related to the family and the lineage, became a powerful way for the gentry to reassert control over the social order. The need to deal with practical problems of local government, which had almost collapsed during the late Ming, also reinforced the tendency to build lineages and kinship solidarity. As interest in lineages grew in the late seventeenth and early eighteenth centuries, disputes over ancestral rites and over the theoretical basis of kinship organisation in turn stimulated scholarly investigations of the classics.

Classical research, more specifically the purist quest to recover ancient ritual forms, and the lineage-building movement became even more closely intertwined in the Han Learning movement of the mid-Qing. Followers of Han Learning considered Cheng-Zhu Confucianism to be based on a corrupt understanding of the classics, and they deployed philological studies to ensure an unperverted understanding of original Confucian ethics. In its criticism of the Cheng-Zhu school, Han Learning strengthened the link between classical research, linguistic purism and ritualistic ethics. The conservative ethics of Han Learning also contributed to the promotion of the ancestral cult and the cult of women's purity, and ritualism came to be regarded by the gentry as the most effective means of excluding heterodox practices. As Chow Kai-wing argues, the rise of ritualism and the proliferation of lineages in late imperial China helped both the imperial state to maintain cultural order and the local élites to enhance their power. Moreover, the gentry's emphasis on proper ceremonies and correct behaviour, on filial piety and loyalty to the monarch reinforced a sense of discipline in which people were expected to abide by correct rules of behaviour rather than seek to understand moral principles for themselves. This emphasis on proper behaviour, self-restraint and ritual practice was not without parallel in a medical discourse which focused on the production of healthy offspring.

THE REGULATION OF DESIRE: SEX, BLOOD AND SEMEN

Many of the medical ideas in late imperial China had already been expressed in the classics of medicine from the early empire and were merely given greater prominence in an approach which underlined the duties of the person in staying healthy. For instance, from its very beginnings medical discourse in China had symbolically linked the person, the state and the cosmos in a holistic vision based on the power of analogy. The medicine of systematic correspondence – a medical epistemology based on the concepts of *yin* and *yang* and the 'five phases' (*wuxing*) dating back to the classical age – wove a network of metaphorical connections between bodily organs and outside substances, multiplied the points of resemblance between microcosmic imbalances in the body and macrocosmic forces in the universe, and accumulated cosmological points of reference that correlated the human body with the political structures of the state.[36] Dual constructions between *yin* and *yang*, hot and cold, wet and dry established sets of analogical relationships between bodily organs, social relations and cosmic

36 For a more detailed analysis, see Paul U. Unschuld, *Medicine in China: A history of ideas*, Berkeley: University of California Press, 1985.

forces: in much the same way as the virtuous rule of the emperor could maintain social order undisturbed by cosmological disorders, the correct behaviour of the individual could ensure good health.

As in many other societies, the appearance of a malformed infant was traditionally interpreted as a warning against society's moral failings. Most babies with severe birth defects were considered to be inauspicious and ill-fated, and were probably destroyed at birth. In conjunction with the political, economic and social changes that characterised the late imperial period, a greater focus on different ways of avoiding the birth of a malformed baby appeared in health manuals. The appearance of a baby who was mentally or physically impaired was seen as not being entirely the result of fate or destiny and was also blamed on the parents themselves. Within this medical discourse, the responsibility of the parents for the health of their descendants started even before conception.

Male and female bodies were correlated to a higher order in medical theory and were thought to be controlled to a significant extent by cosmological forces. Moreover, physiological processes like menstruation and lactation were considered part of a common economy of humours as between male and female. Semen, milk, blood and urine were the interchangeable components of a hierarchy of bodily fluids. Despite an emphasis on similarities between male and female bodies, medical works on female reproductive disorders (*fuke*) emphasised blood (*xue*) to define female difference.[37] Menstrual disorders were elaborated on the basis of *yin* and *yang* categories, and menstruation, represented as a

---

37 See Charlotte Furth, 'Blood, body and gender: Medical images of the female condition in China, 1600–1850', *Chinese Science*, 7 (Dec. 1986), pp. 43–66, and 'Concepts of pregnancy, childbirth, and infancy in Ch'ing dynasty China', *Journal of Asian Studies*, 46, no. 1 (Feb. 1987), pp. 7–35; the author has changed her views in 'Talk on Ming-Qing medicine and the construction of gender', presented at the Institute of History and Philosophy, Taibei, 26 November 1992, a paper which is not for quotation.

key to health and fertility, became a central concern of medicine for women. Menstrual blood was identified as the bodily sign of female generative power. Just as men were told to avoid excessive intercourse and build up their store of semen, health manuals advised women to be continent and to nurture their blood. The reproductive functions of women were increasingly scrutinised, and their bodies were described as intrinsically out of balance, particularly during polluting events like menstruation and pregnancy. Medical specialisations addressed disorders which were thought to be specific to women, children and elderly people, all of whom, in a medical model based on notions of excess and depletion, were represented as having unbalanced and potentially sickly bodies. On the other hand, male reproductive health was defined around the conservation and proper expenditure of semen (*jing*).

If men were gendered as an essential category endowed with powerful desires and enjoined to 'clear the heart and lessen desires' (*qingxin guayu*), women were claimed to be governed by emotions: easily overtaken by anxiety, anger and resentment, they were urged to 'balance the heart and calm the *qi*' (*pingxin dingqi*). Menstrual disorders were a central focus of medical discourse, while regular periods were represented as essential for health and fertility. Health manuals for women noted that infertile women generally suffered from irregular menstruation, which caused a deficiency in either the *qi* or the *xue*. As was common in medieval Europe, particular categories of people were thought to be ruled by different economies of bodily fluids. The distinguished sixteenth-century paediatrician Wan Quan (1488–1578?), one of the most influential followers of the Dongyuan school, noted that fat women (*fei*, meaning fertile in agriculture), when indulging in alcohol and food, remained barren as fat spilled over and blocked the uterus. At the other extreme, thin women (*shou*, meaning infertile in agriculture) suffered from a dry uterus that could not be properly impregnated.[38] Chen Shiduo, a noted Qing doctor, doubted that men who were either excessively corpulent or skinny were capable of healthy reproduction.[39] In a holistic universe which did not make a clear distinction between the cultural and the biological, some social categories of people were seen to be in a constant state of bodily imbalance. Repeating common ideas about socially marginalised women, a local text from Zhejiang province, written in the form of questions and answers, points to the lack of *yang* in young virgins, nuns and widows. Prostitutes, on the other hand, were thought to suffer from a weak *qi*, harmed by excessive intercourse.[40]

Male and female were thus linked through complementary desires, which were to be regulated for the sake of health. In a medical discourse which represented woman's health as dependent upon male sexuality, a lack of intercourse could cause various disorders: Shen Jin'ao (1717–76), a well-known medical writer of Han Learning who also quoted Wan Quan, claimed that 'the menses become deregulated if the female has no intercourse with a male for ten years. Even within a period of ten years she may suffer from deregulated menses if she has pined for intercourse without actually having it.'[41] A notorious writer from Wuxi county in Jiangsu province, Shen Jin'ao only became fully engaged

38 Wan Quan, *Wan shi furenke* (Wan Quan's medicine for women), Wuhan: Hubei renmin chubanshe, 1983, p. 15.

39 Chen Shiduo, *Bianzhenglu* (Writings on medicine), Beijing: Renmin weisheng chubanshe, 1965, p. 374; on the relationship between Fu Shan and Chen Shiduo and the question of authorship, see Li Jinyuan, 'Chen Shiduo ji qi zhuzuo' (Chen Shiduo and his work), *Zhonghua yishi zazhi*, 1988, 18, no. 1, pp. 20–4.

40 *Fuke wenda* (Questions and answers on medicine for women) in Zhu Jianping *et al.* (eds), *Fuke mishu bazhong* (Eight secret books on medicine for women), Beijing: Zhongyi guji chubanshe, 1986, p. 42.

41 Shen Jin'ao, *Fuke yuchi* (The jade rule of medicine for women), orig. 1773, Shanghai: Kexue jishu chubanshe, 1958, p. 14.

in medicine in middle age. Initially trained as a scholar of the classics by Qin Huitian (1702–64) and Gu Donggao (1679–59), two distinguished Han Confucianists who stressed the need to read the classics, he was one of a variety of highly educated scholars who stressed the regulation rather than the suppression of human desires.[42] Like other medical writers, Shen pointed out that nuns and widows suffered amenorrhea when their 'urge' (*yudong*, a term which implies an active impulse) was not satisfied. And in turn, medical treatises emphasised that in the male, infrequent copulation would cause spermatorrhea (*huajing*) and potentially lethal nocturnal emissions (*yijing*).[43] Medical discourse in late imperial China simultaneously endowed the person with desires which were claimed to be a source of generative power, and proposed gender distinctions which were thought to be inherent to male and female bodies. Moreover, medical writers, in particular after the sixteenth century, focused on the inner workings of bodies to the detriment of external influences from the environment or the cosmos. On the other hand, the power of fate, destiny and heavenly retribution was less often highlighted, an indication of the decline in the importance previously attributed to cosmological forces.[44]

42 Xu Ji'ou, 'Shen Jin'ao xiansheng zhuanlüe' (A brief biography of Shen Jin'ao), *Jiangsu zhongyi*, 34 (1963), p. 3.
43 Ming and Qing medical cases provide ample evidence of the widespread concern with nocturnal emissions; see for instance *Song Yuan Ming Qing mingyi lei'an* (Cases from famous physicians from the Song, Yuan, Ming and Qing dynasties), Taibei: Da Zhongguo tushu gongsi, 1971, pp. 42, 70–4 and 102; medical concern with spermatorrhea is clearly expressed, for instance, in Wan Quan, *Wan shi jiachuan yangsheng siyao* (Four essentials of Wan Quan's family notes on nourishing life), Wuhan: Hubei kexue jishu chubanshe, 1984, pp. 43–4, and Chen Shiduo, *Shishi milu* (Secret records of the Stone Chamber), orig. 1687, edn 1805, *juan* 2:18a–20b and 53a–55b.
44 On the decline in belief in cosmology within philosophical circles, see John B. Henderson, *The development and decline of Chinese cosmology*, New York: Columbia University Press, 1984; however, this relative decline does not seem to have undermined common assumptions about the cosmological and moral

Medical disorders were sometimes represented as the result of a pathological agent which could invade the human body, the latter being seen as a fortress to be protected from pathogenic and demonic influences. According to Paul Unschuld,[45] the five phases and the *yin* and *yang* theories of correspondence have not been as important historically as sinologists have assumed. A strong ontological conception of disease – which represented health and ill-health as properties bestowed by nature, by the gods or by other metaphysical entities – has been underestimated in the literature on Chinese medicine. This ontological perspective conceived of pathological agents as intruders needing to be eliminated, and militaristic terminology appeared in Chinese literature in much the same way as was used in European medicine in the pre-bacteriological age. The ontological perspective thrived on notions of 'strength' (*qiang*) and 'weakness' (*ruo*), which were constantly deployed in medical ideas of longevity to qualify bodily substances (blood, semen), types of persons (fat versus thin people, male versus female bodies, urbanites versus farmers) and modes of government: the link between 'strong' citizens and a 'strong' state was made well before the rise of modern nationalism. Appropriating the medical discourse of vitality, the philosopher Yan Yuan even explicitly established a link between physical strength and national power: 'An

---

significance of birth defects in late imperial China; the only direct challenge to such ideas came from Xiong Bolong (1617–69), a fascinating but isolated scholar to whom has been attributed a collection of texts explicitly dismissive of popular stories about sex changes, bearded women and other wondrous phenomena; see Xiong Bolong, *Wuheji* (Philosophical writings), orig. 1794, Beijing: Zhonghua shuju, 1979; see also Wang Mengying, *Guiyanlu* (Writings of Wang Mengying), orig. 1838, repr. Beijing: Zhongyi guji chubanshe, 1987, p. 29.
45 Paul U. Unschuld, 'Epistemological issues and changing legitimation: Traditional Chinese medicine in the twentieth century' in Charles Leslie and Allan Young (eds), *Paths to Asian medical knowledge*, Berkeley: University of California Press, 1992, pp. 44–61.

active body is a strong body, an active home is a strong home, an active country is a strong country.'[46]

Blood (*xue*) in women and semen (*jing*) in men were considered the principal bodily fluids and vital forces determining a person's reproductive health, for the sake of which medical discourse portrayed sex as a potential to be regulated and harnessed. For instance, Wan Quan referred to the *Mencius* in his use of the notion of 'regulation of desires' (*jieyu*). He was the author of numerous health manuals which were frequently reprinted in the seventeenth and eighteenth centuries, and he urged his male readers to monitor carefully a reproductive economy in which finite quantities of semen should be saved in the interests of vitality and posterity: 'The male's semen and the female's blood mingle to generate a foetus. [...] Hence in planting a child, the male should clear his heart, lessen his desire and nurture his semen while the female should balance her heart, calm her *qi* and nurture her blood'.[47] The waste of semen dissipated through excessive intercourse could bring about bodily decay and a decline in generative power. Mingled with female blood, it could lead to new life: health manuals represented human desires as natural impulses, focused on the interior level of the body, and highlighted the responsibility of the person in maintaining health. Only briefly mentioning the existence of larger cosmological forces, Shen Jin'ao also saw conception as the union of male semen and female blood: 'The art of seeking offspring is no more than the nourishment of *jing* in the male and of *xue* in the female.'[48] Conception out of poor blood and weak seed would cause in new-born babies a broken skull, retardation, soft neck, weak limbs, uneven teeth, difficulties in mobility, dis-

---

46 Yan Yuan, *Preservation of Learning* (*Cunxuebian*), translated with an introduction on his life and thought by Mansfield Freeman, Los Angeles: Monumenta Serica, 1972, p. 30.

47 Wan Quan, *Wan shi furenke*, p. 15.

48 Shen Jin'ao, *Fuke yuchi*, p. 1.

colouration of the hair and other defects.[49] Other manuals pointed to the birth of hermaphrodites, cyclops, conjoined twins, and babies with harelips or polydactylia to alert both parents to the importance of reproductive health.[50]

Medical writers directly attributed the innate abilities of offspring to the quality of their parents. Yue Fujia, a seventeenth-century doctor from Lanling county in Jiangsu province who studied the classics before becoming a medical expert, observed that a stupid father and an idiotic mother occasionally succeeded in having many male children, while bright and handsome parents sometimes remained without any children at all. In his experience it also happened that a retarded couple engendered a bright son, while intelligent parents might by accident beget a moron: Yue Fujia believed that the reason for such unexpected variations was to be found in the quality of the father's semen and the mother's blood.[51]

Health manuals dispensed ample advice on how to nourish semen (yangjing) and balance the blood (pingxue) before conception. Assigning responsibility to both the male and the female parent in the production of healthy offspring, medical writers opposed the folk notion that only women were to be held accountable for reproductive abnormalities. One medical text compiled by the monks of the Bamboo Grove monastery, a religious site in Xiaoshan specialising in medicine and issuing publications that became very popular under the Qing,[52] unequivocally attributed duties for the generation of fine seedlings to the male: according to their observations of rich households, concubines who had been

49 Wan Quan, Youke fahui (Exposition of medicine for infants), orig. 1549, Beijing: Renmin weisheng chubanshe, 1963, p. 4.

50 Wang Yanchang, Wangshi, p. 131.

51 Yue Fujia, Miaoyizhai yixue zhengyin zhongzi bian (Yue Fujia's writings on childbirth), orig. 1635, Beijing: Zhongyi guji chubanshe, 1986, p. 5.

52 See Liao Yuqun, 'Xiaoshan zhulinsi nüke kaolüe' (Investigation of the work on medicine for women of the Bamboo Grove monastery in Xiaoshan), Zhonghua yishi zazhi, 1986, 16, no. 3, pp. 159–61.

purchased on the basis of their fertility would not necessarily be impregnated: 'Why is it that some become pregnant in
one case and not in the other? It is because the responsibility for the generation of offspring rests entirely with the
male.'[53] The male bestowed, the female received, much as
the seed was planted on fertile soil. Metaphors taken from
rice cultivation supported a protean vision of human conception in which the quality of offspring could be nurtured
and improved at every stage: the selection of seed, the
preparation of soil, the use of fertilisers, even the elimination of sickly seedlings were common practices in agriculture, and these found an echo in medical descriptions of
human reproduction. Contrary to some European countries, metaphors taken from animal breeding were not
significant in medical discourse.

Shen Jin'ao listed five ways of strengthening seed, namely
the regulation of sexual intercourse and the avoidance of
sexual fatigue, anger, and the intake of alcohol and spicy
foods.[54] In a holistic universe governed by correlative thinking, any emotional imbalance could leave a physical lesion,
while uncontrolled passions would leave their mark on the
body. Anger could hurt the liver, which was responsible for
the regulation of fluids, while excessive sexual activity
would harm the kidney. As in eighteenth-century Europe,
somatic reasons were invoked to explain sexual intemper-
ance: in England, for instance, spicy food, excessive wine,
aphrodisiacs or genital irritation were thought to trigger
desire, and the consequences of excess were primarily
depicted in terms of physical disorders, such as exhaustion,
infertility, baldness and premature death.[55] Similarly, alcohol
in China was seen as agitating the blood and weakening the

53 Zhulinsi sengren, *Zhulinsi nüke erzhong* (Two texts on medicine for women
by the Bamboo Grove monastery), orig. 1786, Beijing: Zhongyi guji chubanshe, 1993, p. 294.
54 Shen Jin'ao, *Fuke yuchi*, p. 1.
55 Roy Porter, 'Love, sex, and madness in eighteenth-century England', *Social
Research*, no. 53 (1986), pp. 211–42.

semen. The consequences of excess were dire: weak persons who had carefully nourished their blood for several months could waste it in a single evening's bout. Spicy food, in turn, was considered detrimental to the generation of semen, which could only be invigorated by balanced and mildly flavoured meals.[56]

According to ideas comparable to those current in early modern Europe, sex was seen as a normal desire which should be satisfied in moderation – neither too much nor too little. The denial of sex in Europe was seen as unnatural and possibly leading to physical disorders such as chlorosis or hysteria. Sex, as Roy Porter has asserted, was not intimately linked with alienation of the mind in traditional medico-moral discourse.[57] Similarly, in the opinion of late Ming and Qing medical writers, excessive sexual intercourse was an important reason for male reproductive problems. Offspring conceived by degraded semen would suffer from five kinds of maldevelopment (*wuchi*) or five kinds of flabbiness (*wuruan*).[58] Using medical examples to illustrate his exhortations for a disciplined approach to sexual intercourse, Yue Fujia invoked the case of a young and healthy man whose wife did not bear him any children. All the doctors he had consulted blamed infertility on his wife and advised him to take a concubine, but examining his pulse, Yue established that he suffered from heat-evil and depletion of semen due to endless drinking bouts, gambling into the early hours of the morning and constant intercourse with women. After the young man had followed his strict

56 Shen Jin'ao, *Fuke yuchi*, p. 1.
57 Roy Porter, *Mind-forg'd manacles: A history of madness in England from the Restoration to the Regency*, London: Penguin Books, 1990, p. 202.
58 On growth tardiness in Ming and Qing medical texts, see Hsiung Ping-chen, 'Chuantong Zhongguo yijie dui chengzhang yu fayu xianxiang de taolun' (Debates about growth and development in traditional Chinese medicine), *Guoli Taiwan shifan daxue lishi xuebao*, no. 20 (July 1992), pp. 27–40.

instructions against sexual excesses, his wife was successfully impregnated and later conceived a son.[59]

In a holistic conception of the body, medical theories related all organs to each other and rarely discussed them separately. Blood as well as semen were 'excreted' in one and the same movement in a common economy of bodily fluids which had to remain in balance if the person was to stay healthy. For women, failure to menstruate was interpreted as a sign of bodily disorder, and the purging of excess blood was claimed to be inherently health-maintaining. As much as purges, emetics and other remedies were used to re-establish the menstrual flow in women, aphrodisiac products said to enhance reproductive vitality were prescribed for men. Many health manuals, indicating the widespread use of medications in late imperial China, warned against such products. Remedies to replenish the yin (*ziyin*), tonics to invigorate the *qi* (*yangqi*), prescriptions to nourish the kidney (*bushen*), medications to give tone to the blood (*buxue*): such medical therapies to achieve vitality proliferated throughout the late imperial period.

Medical authors of the Ming and Qing warned against abuse of tonics and indulgence in aphrodisiacs. Spermatorrhea (*huajing*), premature ejaculation (*zaoxie*) and nocturnal emissions (*mengyi*) were some of the pathological categories constructed by medical discourse in order to enforce a message of restraint. For instance, Yue Fujia deplored the abuse of warming medications (*reyao*) that caused *yang* hyperactivity (*kangyang*), since it would heighten sexual pleasure for a while but lead in the long term to a pathological depletion of semen. He noted that many highly-placed officials who used warming drugs suffered from huge quantities of blood in the urine (*niaoxue*), pus in the scrotum (*nangyong*) and lung abscesses (*feiyong*), three lethal disorders caused by heat-evil.[60] In the dangerous pursuit of vitality, a disciplined

59 Yue, *Miaoyizhai*, pp. 11–12.
60 Yue, *Miaoyizhai*, pp. 11–12.

practise of sexual intercourse and a balanced approach to food had the potential to increase a person's generative power, prolonging life and multiplying one's descendants. By contrast, as health manuals continuously warned, indulgence, abuse and excess would turn a potent weapon into a malevolent force, leading to a depletion of vital forces, provoking a waste of bodily substances, inviting debilitating disorders, and even leading to early death. Death of the self and death of the lineage: according to Wang Yanchang, aphrodisiacs (chunfangyao) were destructive and capable of killing a male and extinguishing a line of descent.[61]

THE DANGERS OF EXCESS: MARITAL HARMONY AND COSMOLOGICAL CONSONANCE

'To the one who seeks descendants, the selection of a female is just what the selection of soil is to the planter,' intoned the monks of the Bamboo Grove monastery, who issued two texts on female reproductive disorders which were widely disseminated in the late eighteenth century. 'One can hardly expect rice and wheat to grow on gravel: how could one hope that a women of poor blessings would bear a son?'[62] Like the prescriptions that had marked the bedchamber genre, the physical and moral qualities of the female partner were listed by medical writers in some detail. However, the age of the two partners seemed to be of greater concern to different authors. If intercourse between two healthy partners could lead to the birth of a sturdy child, some medical publications pointed to the dangerous consequences of early marriage. The male should wait till thirty and the female till twenty – ages at which their yin and yang were fully formed. The eighteenth-century classi-

61 Wang Yanchang, Wangshi yicun (Writings of Wang Yanchang), orig. 1871, Hangzhou: Jiangsu kexue jishu chubanshe, 1983, p. 50.
62 Zhulinsi, Nüke, p. 293.

cist Wu Qian cautioned that before full maturity, copulation could cause premature leaking of *yin qi* (*yinqi zaoxie*), leading to infertility or to weak offspring.[63]

If human procreation was explained as a fusion of paternal semen and maternal blood, the propitious convergence of cosmic movements remained paramount. The sections of medical treatises concerning human reproduction generally opened with a statement on the cosmological implications of conception and pointed to the interdependence between Heaven and Earth and sexual intercourse. Correlations between the lunar and menstrual cycles were established, linking the human body to a macrocosm: 'From the new moon to the full moon, when menstrual blood circulates and follows its course, conception is easy and offspring will be long-lived, as the moon gradually waxes; from the full moon to the last day of the lunar month, when menstrual blood circulates or deviates from its period, it will be difficult for the foetus to take shape, and often as the moon gradually wanes, offspring will come to a premature end.'[64] The gathering of the generative forces of Heaven and Earth was signalled by the end of the menstrual cycle, a privileged moment when the woman 'appears drunken or mad, as if she cannot resist the desire to have intercourse'.[65] The authors of the medical texts published by the Bamboo Grove monastery also thought that this was the best time for conception, marked by an extreme yearning for pleasure even in animals: 'Just before becoming pregnant, the female cat and dog mew and howl furiously and run around.'[66]

A system of taboos based on belief in a correlation between macrocosm and microcosm governed sexual intercourse. The resonance between the female body and heav-

63 Wu Qian, *Fuke xinfa yaojue* (Essentials of personal experiences in medicine for women), orig. 1742, repr. in *Yizong jinjian* (The golden mirror of medicine), orig. 1749, Beijing: Renmin weisheng chubanshe, 1988, p. 45.
64 Wan Quan, *Wan shi furenke*, p. 16.
65 Wu Qian, *Fuke xinfa*, p. 46.
66 Zhulinsi, *Nüke*, p. 298.

enly body could be thrown out of balance by a natural cata-strophe. By analogy, any cosmological disruption during the coupling of male and female could leave a physical lesion on future offspring: according to the popular health manuals which circulated in late imperial China, eclipses, thunder, storms, floods and earthquakes could engender deaf, mute, blind or retarded children. Tang Qianqing's *Dasheng yaozhi* (1762) explained how, by a similar principle, favourable weather conditions contributed to a peaceful environment propitious for conception.[67] Particular spaces like temples, shrines, graves, kitchens and latrines were also proscribed: they were said to create a negative state of mind and power-ful emotions that could influence the health of offspring.

If human conception had to be in accord with broader cosmological forces – sophisticated almanacs indicated favourable and unfavourable days – the medicine of system-atic correspondence demanded that great attention be paid to diet, emotions and even gestures, all of which were preg-nant with a power of resonance which could be detrimental to foetal health: a child conceived out of rape was of a vio-lent disposition, while the descendants of drunken parents were marked by mental retardation: 'Scholars and govern-ment officials in the Jiangnan region often wallow in women and song. When taking a wife or concubine, they search for young and pretty ones, although the children they conceive are all weak and disease-ridden, dying at an early age. These gentlemen even enter the bedroom com-pletely drunk, with their minds dazed and confused, hence their offspring are slow-witted.'[68]

The concern for moderation and the necessity of caution became even more vital for pregnant women, whose bodies lived in close affinity with the environment. Medical writers

67 Tang Qianqing, *Dasheng yaozhi* (Essentials on successful childbirth), orig. 1762, 1847 edn, *juan* 1:2a.
68 Yu Tan, *Xishang futan* (Talks on the mat), Shanghai: Shangwu yinshuguan, 1936, p. 16.

railed against sexual intercourse during pregnancy, portraying the newly-conceived embryo as a vulnerable substance needing protection from further 'charges' and 'assaults' (*chongji*). Wan Quan intoned: 'In ancient times, women lived in separate quarters and did not have sexual intercourse with their husbands after they became pregnant, hence they had no difficulties during delivery. Many of their children were born virtuous and suffered from few disorders. Today, people know no restrictions and indulge in their desires to their hearts' content. There are those who move the foetus's *qi* and cause it to abort, there are foetuses that stiffen and are hard to deliver, [...] there are children born with numerous disorders, some entirely covered with smallpox pustules: all are the result of excessive sexual congress.'[69] Some authors acknowledged that observing total abstinence during pregnancy was difficult, but insisted on the strict regulation of sexual desire, since any lecherous excesses (*yinyu zhi guo*) led inevitably to miscarriage, foetal disorders and even the death of the offspring. Impetuous intercourse could dislodge an embryo which had not yet been identified: it would be discharged from the womb like any other vaginal fluid without the couple even suspecting its existence.

Moral exhortations and medical warnings converged in a discourse which focused on the dangers of excess. The power of analogy somehow linked blind indulgence in the pleasures of the flesh to a less blissful form of ignorance, as frequent sexual congress unwittingly led to a vicious circle of conceptions and miscarriages: 'The embryo conceived yesterday is aborted today without anybody knowing.'[70] In a similar vein, it was noted that those who married prostitutes were often left without descendants, simply because the wombs of such women had been spoiled by frequent

---

69 Wan Quan, *Wan shi furenke*, p. 20.
70 Zhulinsi, *Nüke*, p. 301.

miscarriages and were too slippery to retain the embryo.[71] A strict separation of the sexes during pregnancy was enjoined by health manuals in order to ensure the preservation of the foetus;[72] even cats and dogs knew the dangers of sexual excess and refrained from copulating after conception.[73]

Health manuals also recommended extreme caution in posture and movement as one went about one's everyday's existence. These were to be closely monitored in the interest of future offspring. A pregnant woman should not ascend to a high place (*denggao*) or stretch out her arm to reach a high object. Regular movement, on the other hand, promoted the circulation of *xue* and *qi* and would ease the actual birth. Contrasting the frugal mores of sturdy peasants to the degenerate habits of an idle gentry, Wan Quan did not spare women who spent their time in leisurely pursuits. Lack of exertion would lead to difficulty in giving birth, and pregnant women should walk and sit upright.[74] Other medical writers pointed out that the muscles and bones were strengthened through regular exercise; as one could see, peasant women who tilled the fields gave birth easily.[75]

Basing their reasoning on the power of analogy, medical writers saw diet as a foundation of reproductive health. Symbolic meanings were assigned to food products, weaving a close network of correlations between macrocosm and microcosm. Food could be health-giving or life-endangering: the condition of harelip in the new-born baby was induced by the consumption of rabbit meat, while sheep's blood could cause albino eyes. Many health manuals extended their dietary restrictions to crabs, tortoises, spar-

71 Ibid.
72 Li Changke, *Taichan husheng pian* (On childbirth and the protection of life), orig. 1798, 1862 edn, *juan* 1, pp. 16b–18b.
73 Huang Tizhai, *Taichan jiyao* (Essentials of childbirth), orig. 1756, 1839 edn, *juan* 1, p. 2a.
74 Wan Quan, *Wan shi furenke*, p. 21.
75 Zhulinsi, *Nüke*, p. 135.

rows and shellfish, as well as spices like ginger, pepper and garlic: beyond its heating properties, ginger could cause polydactylia in the foetus. According to one nineteenth-century manual, weird combinations of food, such as eel with frog, could lead to a variety of strange deformities in the foetus.[76] Mild flavours (dan), avoiding both cold and heat, would nourish the foetus with a clear qi and prevent the child from contracting diseases. Women of his day, Wan Quan intimated, carelessly indulged in all sorts of flavours and dishes. Failure to restrain the appetite would harm the spleen and stomach and in turn induce abortion. Also, indiscriminate mixing of hot and cold food would give rise to various medical conditions. The medicine of systematic correspondence established close correlations between the five flavours and the five organs: bitter (ku) the heart (xin), sweet (gan) the spleen (pi), acrid (xin) the lungs (fei), salt (xian) the kidney (shen), and sour (suan) harmed the stomach (wei). A warning was given that excessive consumption of alcoholic drinks would induce promiscuity (luanxing) and cause a lecherous child to be engendered. The semen of the male would become mixed up (luanjing) and the foetus would suffer from a variety of disorders.[77]

In a holistic universe governed by somatisation, the pregnant woman was at the centre of a fragile system of correlations in which the slightest emotional disturbance could bring about a physical lesion. Excessive joy caused damage to the heart, anger harmed the liver, while fear destroyed the kidney: physical retribution followed every variety of emotional excess. A discourse of restraint depicted the consequences of excess in stark medical terms, and failure to keep to the requirements of moderation brought about malformations in the foetus, which was born 'blind, deaf and mute, retarded and epileptic'.[78] The affective economy of a

76 Yongsitang zhuren, Taichan hebi (Two books on childbirth), orig. 1862 edn., juan 1, p. 3ab.

77 Zhulinsi, Nüke, pp. 137 and 296.

78 Wan Quan, Wan shi furenke, p. 21.

woman in gestation was capable of releasing violent passions, generating emotional impulses, and falling into fits of
anger, and thus demanded strict supervision. If miscarriage
was like 'the fruit that drops from a withered twig, the
flower that falls from a shrivelled vine', strong emotions and
fits of anger could dislodge the foetus 'as wind shakes a
tree'.[79] Violent anger, in particular the use of evil words,
was to be avoided, since it would harm the *qi* and the blood
which nourishes the foetus: disturbed blood could agitate
the foetus or, alternatively, angry *qi* (*nuqi*) could enter it and
it would consequently suffer from phlegm at birth.[80] Other
treatises on medicine for women, which circulated at
provincial levels, also stressed that irregular menses were the
main cause of medical disorders in women, although emotions such as lust, hatred, jealousy and melancholy were the
'deep roots' of disorders which occurred ten times more
often in women than in men.[81] The social anxieties aroused
by female emotions haunted the medical imagination,
structured marital relations and even governed domestic life,
as any irritation was claimed to have repercussions on the
foetus.

   These medical injunctions were sometimes invoked
under the name of foetal education (*taijiao*), although evidence for its popularity in Ming and Qing medical dis-

79 Shan Nanshan, *Taichan zhinan* (Guide to childbirth), orig. 1856, Shanghai:
Dadong shuju, 1936, p. 27.
80 Shen Jin'ao, *Fuke yuchi*, p. 56.
81 *Jiachuan nüke jingyan zhaiqi* (Strange passages from passed-on experiences in
medicine for women) in Zhu Jianping *et al.* (eds), *Fuke mishu bazhong* (Eight secret
books on medicine for women), Beijing: Zhongyi guji chubanshe, 1986, p. 170.
82 Foetal education (*taijiao*) was not especially emphasised in the eighteenth
century, according to Charlotte Furth ('Concepts of pregnancy', pp. 14–15),
although it was clearly invoked by a number of medical treatises; moreover, the
idea of maternal impression (*ganshou muqi*) was important in sixteenth-century
paediatric literature before it disappeared in the seventeenth century, according
to Xiong Bingzhen, 'Chuantong Zhongguo yijie dui changcheng yu fayu
xianxiang de taolun' (Debates about growth and development in traditional

course is contradictory.[82] Most health manuals which focused on human reproduction simply quoted from older texts, for instance the *Lienüzhuan*: 'The eyes will see no evil colours, the ears will hear no evil sounds, the mouth will speak no evil words: this is the meaning of foetal education.'[83] Whether foetal education was directly invoked or not, all medical theories played on the importance of correct behaviour in pregnant women for the sake of healthy off-spring. The great emphasis which medical authors laid on restraint and propriety corresponded largely to the importance on self-cultivation by Confucian purists under the Qing. Zhang Boxing (1652–1725), the incorruptible governor of Jiangsu province and austere follower of Cheng-Zhu Confucianism,[84] wrote of foetal education and correct behaviour in pregnant women in a preface to a compilation which has not survived.[85]

The belief that the strict observance of proper rituals and formal rules of behaviour could nurture individual wisdom even among common people was widespread among Confucianists, who attempted to impart their knowledge to the widest possible public. Following ortho-dox tradition, Zhang Boxing also compiled a text on the education of young children, detailing all the rites to be followed, such as washing and combing, dressing, formal bowing, kneeling, standing, sitting, walking and talking, eating and drinking, serving elders at table and receiving guests. Although the origin of such written family injunctions can be traced back to the *Classic of Rites* (*Liji*), they

Chinese medicine), *Guoli Taiwan shifan daxue lishi xuebao*, no. 20 (July 1992), pp. 27–40.

83 *Taiping yulan* (Song encyclopaedia), 'Lienüzhuan', Taipei: Xinxing shuju, 1959, p. 1694 (360:8).

84 A short note on Zhang Boxing appears in Jonathan D. Spence, 'Collapse of a purist' in *Chinese roundabout: Essays in history and culture*, New York: W.W. Norton, 1992, pp. 124–31.

85 Zhang Boxing, *Zhengyi tang wenji* (Collected works of Zhang Boxing), Shanghai: Shangwu yinshuguan, 1937, no. 62, *juan* 87, pp. 6a–7b.

became especially popular during the Qing throughout the populated cities of the coastal regions but particularly in the Jiangnan region. For instance, the *Family Instructions* (*Jiating jianghua*) of 1837 prescribed the proper behaviour to be followed by young boys and girls during the different periods of life. At a very early stage, the girl had to learn the use of her body: how to sit and stand, and how to bow. From the age of five or six onwards, she was to be confined inside the home instead of roaming about outside. At ten she would be forbidden to play with boys. The proper etiquette to be observed with guests was taught at the age of twelve or thirteen. Having reached sixteen, she was forbidden to gaze outside the house, to get up late, to talk or laugh loudly, to read lewd verses and fiction, or to gamble or play dominoes: she was now considered ready for marriage and motherhood.

These family instructions were printed on paper of poor quality and written in vernacular Chinese; as with the medical publications analysed here, they probably ended up in the hands of numerous Jiangnan shopkeepers, merchants, doctors, teachers and artisans.[86] Educate in order to regulate – this could well have been the motto of many a Confucian scholar, as the idea of self-cultivation spread among the urban public of the coastal region. The education of a person according to the rules of foetal education was deemed to start at the very moment of conception.

THE TORMENTS OF IMAGINATION: MATERNAL IMPRINTS AND GHOSTLY FOETUSES

In early modern England, anxiety about the 'dangerous prevalence of imagination' was expressed by Hobbes to

---

86 See Joseph P. McDermott, 'The Chinese domestic bursar', *Ajia bunka kenkyu*, no. 2 (Nov. 1990), p. 284; I am grateful to Joseph McDermott for a copy of parts of the original of the *Family Instructions*.

Samuel Johnson.[87] In the eighteenth century, the common belief that the imagination of a pregnant woman could deform her foetus came to be widely discussed in medical and philosophical circles throughout Europe, a debate closely related to fears of a transgression of clear boundaries between body and mind. Based on a dualistic vision of human identity, divided into a material body and a spiritual mind, images of monstrosity were deployed to explore the problematic nature of the self as a coherent and autonomous category.[88] In China, where boundaries between the psychological and the physiological were thought of as permeable, 'imagination' did not exist as a powerful category specific to the mind, although mental anxiety was interpreted as one of several emotions which could lead to bodily disorders. Mental anxiety (si) could trigger a burning lust in unsatisfied women. Chen Shiduo observed that they could suddenly 'go mad' and, driven by excessive yearning (simu), copulate with any male; among the medical disorders that flowed from these sexual cravings was epilepsy (dianxian).[89] Characterised as a passive category in opposition to the more active endowment of men, women were said to pine for the roborant absorption of male secretions. For Li Chan,

87 D.F. Bond, '"Distrust" of imagination in English neoclassicism', *Philological Quarterly*, no. 14 (1937), pp. 54–69; D.F. Bond, 'The neoclassical psychology of the imagination', *English Literature and History*, no. 4 (1937), pp. 245–64; J. Engell, *The creative imagination*, Cambridge, MA: Harvard University Press, 1981.

88 See Paul-Gabriel Boucé, 'Imagination, pregnant women, and monsters in eighteenth-century England and France' in G.S. Rousseau and Roy Porter (eds), *Sexual underworlds of the Enlightenment*, Manchester: Manchester University Press, 1987, pp. 87–100; Philip K. Wilson, '"Out of sight, out of mind?": The Daniel Turner-James Blondel dispute over the power of the maternal imagination', *Annals of Science*, no. 49 (1992), pp. 159–97; Marie – Hélène Huet, *Monstrous imagination*, Cambridge, MA: Harvard University Press, 1993; Dennis Todd, *Imagining monsters: Miscreations of the self in eighteenth-century England*, University of Chicago Press, 1995.

89 Chen Shiduo, *Shishi milu* (Secret records of the Stone Chamber), orig. 1687, 1805 edn, *juan* 1, p. 41a.

a sixteenth-century physician from Jiangxi province, merely thinking (*si*) of men could harm the heart, deplete the spleen and exhaust the kidney of young girls under the age of twenty; this was a wasting disorder which might be difficult to cure.[90] According to others, unmarried girls, neglected concubines, lonely widows and solitary nuns who could not satisfy their sexual desires would 'feel aggrieved beyond expression', as the flames of fancy would lead to amenorrhea or even consumptive disorders (*laozhai*).[91]

In addition to the capacity of female sexual desire to induce bodily imbalances, a woman's mind could quite literally engender a monster. It was a medium by which harmful influences could be transmitted, rather than the repository of a dangerous but independent imagination. It imposed strict restrictions. 'After conception, one should not go to the theatre or look at ghostly and monstrous images (*guiguai xingxiang*)'; this message was frequently repeated in health manuals during the Qing.[92] Wan Quan called the relationship between maternal image and foetal shape 'external impression and internal response' (*waixiang er neigan*).[93] The shape of the foetus was indeterminate and underwent change according to the objects seen by the mother, who should avoid looking at ugly and deformed people. Wan Quan himself observed how women who often watched puppet theatre and monkey shows during pregnancy later gave birth to children with simian features. As the foetus gradually took shape during the first three months after conception, it could hear via its mother (*sui mu tingwen*), who should take care regularly to listen to

90 Li Chan, *Yixue rumen* (Elementary medicine), orig. 1575, quoted in Shen Jin'ao, *Fuke yuchi*, p. 23.

91 Shen Jin'ao, *Fuke yuchi*, pp. 23–4.

92 Huang Tizhai, *Taichan jiyao* (Essentials of childbirth), orig. 1756, 1839 edn, *juan* 1, p. 2a.

93 Wan Quan, *Yuying mijue* (Secrets on child-rearing), orig. 1549, repr. in *Mingdai Wan Mizhai erke quanshu* (The collected works on medicine for children of Wan Quan), Beijing: Zhongyi guji chubanshe, 1991, pp. 36–9.

good words, request people to read books aloud to others and explain the rules of propriety and music (*liyue*), and avoid hearing evil talk. Encouragingly, Yan Chunxi, a government official in Hebei province, wrote that listening to scholarly pieces of work might even assist in begetting a son.[94] The children born to women who followed these simple rules would live long and be sincere, virtuous and intelligent; failure to follow them would result in stupid and vulgar offspring being born. Many health manuals used the notion of 'external impression and internal response' to impress on their audience the view that good literature should be read to the mother in order to nurture an upright child during the third month of pregnancy.

In a symbolic universe governed by somatisation, excessive emotions could present a danger to reproductive health. It was endlessly repeated that monstrous images and strange objects would frighten the mother and induce epilepsy in the foetus (*dianxian*). According to Zhang Yaosun, a government official and medical expert of Jiangsu province, simply looking at 'monstrous animals and strange birds' or at 'violent and sinister shapes' was an action full of danger, as the mind of the mother could be shocked to the point of inducing a deformity in the foetus.[95] Inspired by the Dongyuan school, Wang Kentang's widely read work on childbirth suggested that people with deformed features or misshapen appearance should be avoided because the shape (*xing*) of the foetus remained malleable during the first three months of pregnancy.[96] The *Essentials of childbirth*, a popular eighteenth-century manual compiled by Ke Jia, went so far

94 Yan Chunxi, *Taichan xinfa* (Personal experience in childbirth), orig. 1730, 1824 edn., *juan* 1, 10b–11a; on Yan Chunxi, see Guo Junshuang and Tian Daihua, 'Yan Chunxi yu *Taichan xinfa*' (Yan Chunxi and his book on childbirth), *Zhonghua yishi zazhi*, 1990, 20, no. 3, pp. 180–3.

95 Zhang Yaosun, *Chanyunji* (On childbirth), orig. 1830, Shanghai: Dadong shuju, 1936, p. 15.

96 Wang Kentang, *Chanbao baiwen* (A hundred questions on childbirth), orig. 1559, 1602 edn, first part, pp. 5a–8a.

as to prohibit women from looking at wild animals, in particular tortoises, snakes and rabbits, for fear of producing offspring with bestial features.[97] The popular *Dashengbian* (Book on successful childbirth), reprinted more than eighty times, added 'murderous and evil' scenes (*zaisha xiongwu*) to its list of ominous occurrences from which pregnant women should avert their eyes.[98] Similar injunctions can be found in many other health manuals, although Shen Jin'ao, a prolific author of medical books, regretted that they sometimes failed to convince common people: medical exhortations should 'hit the eye and stir the heart' (*chumu jingxin*) of the reader.[99] The power of words to fill the heart of a reader with dread was comparable to the ability of images to shake the minds of pregnant women, participating in an ambiguous discourse which highlighted the power of analogy in a universe of systematic correspondences where a psychological sensation was easily transformed into a physical lesion.

The morbidity of the female mind was attested to by medical cases. At the end of the sixteenth century, it was reported how a family raising turtles conceived several rickety children with a tortoise breast (*guixiong*, also called *jixiong*, 'chicken breast') characterised by a prominent sternum.[100] The mother had while pregnant absorbed an evil *qi* from the turtles. Another unfortunate couple, residing next to a temple with clay figures, gave birth to a hideous child with a couple of fleshy excrescences on its head and two high nostrils, thus bearing an uncanny resemblance to the malevolent spirit yaksha, whose image must have imposed

97 Ke Jia, *Baochan jiyao* (Essentials of childbirth) in *Hecuan dashengpian baochan jiyao* (Two medical works on successful childbirth), orig. 1779 edn, p. 5b.

98 *Dashengbian* (Book on successful childbirth), orig. 1715, Shanghai: Foxue shuju, 1934, pp. 11–12.

99 Shen Jin'ao, *Fuke yuchi*, p. 56.

100 Jiang Guan, *Mingyi lei'an* (Classified medical cases from famous physicians), orig. 1591, 1770 edn, Taibei: Hongye shuju, 1971, p. 335.

itself on to the foetus.[101] Others asserted that intercourse with a deity during a nightly visit to a temple could lead to a swollen belly. In one case, an impregnated woman expelled nearly two litres of swarming tadpoles after the use of an abortifacient (duotaiyao).[102]

Excessive longing for sexual intercourse could even cause an alien spirit to take possession of the womb. Ghostly foetuses regularly appeared in medical cases throughout the Qing. Xu Dachun, a great classicist who advocated a return to the medical classics, reported the case of a woman in her early thirties who suffered from amenorrhea for eight to nine months and had a swollen belly. Drawing on demonology, which was sometimes integrated into the medicine of systematic correspondence under the Ming and Qing,[103] Xu diagnosed a disorder of the liver and the spleen induced by the presence of an evil spirit (guisui) that had impregnated itself upon the imagination of the patient. After being given a medical infusion, she lost a huge quantity of foul blood and filthy fluids as well as an afterbirth containing a clot of blood. A closer examination of this misshapen lump of flesh revealed the imprint of a ghostly face. This strange event was duly put on record by Xu Dachun.[104] Wei Zhixiu reported the case of a woman possessed by a spirit who after a pregnancy lasting fourteen months delivered an inanimate object shaped like a goldfish.[105] On more common cultural terrain, health manuals like the Book of Secrets on Medicine for Women also discoursed at length about spectral foetuses (guitai), the result of an imaginary sexual encounter with a spirit. Conceived by an unbridled imagination which inflamed

101 Ibid.
102 Sun Zhihong, Jianming yigou (Concise essentials of medicine), orig. 1629, Beijing: Renmin weisheng chubanshe, 1984, p. 406.
103 See Unschuld, Medicine in China, p. 218
104 Xu Dachun, Nüke yi'an (Medical cases in medicine for women), orig. 1764, repr. in Xu Dachun yishu quanji (Complete medical works of Xu Dachun), Beijing: Renmin weisheng chubanshe, 1988, p. 1873.
105 Jiang Guan, Mingyi lei'an, p. 331.

the 'ministerial fires', white secretions were retained in the womb and combined with menstrual blood to form a monstrous foetus. The blood clot which colonised the womb for months on end symbolised both the power and the sterility of female imagination.[106]

Monstrous shapes could be conceived even without the help of a libidinous imagination. For instance, a woman ten months pregnant was said to have given birth to half a bucket full of crawling white worms. Although semen and blood had successfully coagulated inside her womb, a lack of vital energy (*yuanqi*) had precluded its transformation into a human foetus. The power of analogy was such that it could bring about a metamorphosis, since a combination of corrupt substances had spontaneously generated worms, 'comparable to filthy canals and ditches which stagnate and engender all sorts of insects'. A medical case of this nature was characterised as an inauspicious event, highlighting the close association of vermin with guilt; the woman was reported to have died within a month.[107] As in medieval Europe, inert matter could be transformed into live creatures, and insects could be born from putrefaction and evil humidity. When humidity became entirely putrid it caused a disorder of the skin, according to the fourteenth-century royal surgeon Henri de Mondeville, but when it received the vital spirit it could generate small animals: as in China, the retention of menstrual blood in women of 'sanguine temperament' was thought to generate worms.[108] In a holistic universe, the belief in spontaneous generation was closely linked to the power of analogy, as inanimate matter was metamorphosed into animate creatures and organic dis-

106 *Fuke mishu* (Book of secrets on medicine for women) in Zhu Jianping *et al.* (eds), *Fuke mishu bazhong* (Eight secret books on medicine for women), Beijing: Zhongyi guji chubanshe, 1986, pp. 112–13.

107 Jiang Guan and Wei Zhixiu, *Xu mingyi lei'an* (More classified medical cases from famous physicians), orig. 1770 edn, Taibei: Hongye shuju, 1971, p. 605.

108 Marie-Christine Pouchelle, *The body and surgery in the Middle Ages*, New Brunswick, NJ: Rutgers University Press, 1990, pp. 169–70.

orders could subtly mutate into an infestation. Worms and insects were born of the putrefaction of bodies and the decomposition of earth; an example of this was the widow whose vagina engendered insects, became corrupt and rotted away, gradually turning into vermin who gnawed at her entrails to finally grow into a myriad of red worms, each the size of a thumb.[109]

EPILOGUE: LINEAGE, 'RACE' AND REPRODUCTION DURING THE LATE QING

In this chapter we have noted that the rise of ritualism and the consolidation of lineages in late imperial China was helpful both to the imperial state in maintaining cultural order and to the local élites in enhancing their power. In resonance with the rise of political conservatism under the Qing, medical knowledge which emphasised the need for individuals to restrain their desires for the sake of the lineage was promoted by involvement of the gentry in medical publications.

Besides these trends, demographic pressure and political tensions under the Qing also contributed to the rise of a conservative philosophy of sexual restraint. Although a conception of population control had already emerged in the writings of Hong Liangji (1746–1809), a scholar who developed ideas of overpopulation five years before Thomas Malthus' *Essay on the principle of population* (1798),[110] the most astonishing vision of sexual restraint was expressed in the privacy of a secret journal by Wang Shiduo (1802–89), preceptor of the Imperial Academy and adviser to the gov-

109 Jiang Guan, *Mingyi lei'an*, p. 478.
110 On demographic thought and the emergence of 'population' as an analytical category, see Frank Dikötter, *Sex, culture and modernity in China: Medical science and the construction of sexual identities in the early Republican period*, London: Hurst; Honolulu: University of Hawaii Press; Hong Kong University Press, 1995, chapter 4, pp. 102–21.

ernor of Hubei province.[111] Here he outlined a theory of
state power based on the limitation of births and the regulation of sexuality. In this journal which he wrote during the
turbulent years of the Taiping rebellion (1850–64) he
observed: 'There are too many women, hence there are too
many people; because there are too many people, they are
poor and there is not enough available land to support
them.' Distressed by the growing number of paupers, he
proclaimed: 'Heaven has its material for slaughter. Among
animals they are the sheep, the pigs, the chickens and the
ducks; among humans they are the short and puny, ugly,
mean-eyed, short-stepped, garrulous, effeminate and stupid
people.'[112] Wang confided to his journal that taxes should
be imposed on the female population to implement a thorough infanticide policy: all female children born of poor
parents and sons who were physically abnormal or did not
have handsome features should be drowned; temples, nun-
neries, 'institutes for virgin women' and 'halls of chastity'
should be constructed in large numbers; people should be
encouraged to become monks or nuns or remain unmarried; and women with one living child should be compelled
to take abortifacient drugs to terminate their pregnancies.
Wang Shiduo was certainly a marginal thinker, but he
expressed more explicitly a concern which would surface
periodically in the writings of other nineteenth-century
scholars; he focused on the regulation of reproductive
behaviour for the sake of the social organism. It was from a
concern within families over the continuation of the lineage
that human sexuality and reproduction gradually emerged as
a public domain linked to the strength of the country.

The Taiping rebellion, during which Wang Shiduo wrote
his diary, was an era of popular unrest marked by a consoli-

111 Frank Dikötter, 'The limits of benevolence: Wang Shiduo (1802–1889)
and population control', *Bulletin of the School of Oriental and African Studies*, 55,
no. 1 (February 1992), pp. 110–15.
112 Wang Shiduo, *Wang Huiweng yibing riji* (Diary of Wang Shiduo), Taibei:
Wenhai chubanshe, 1967, p. 145.

dation of the cult of patrilineal descent, and this formed the centre of a broad movement of social reform that had emphasised the family and the lineage since the collapse of the Ming. Considerable friction arose between lineages throughout the nineteenth century in response to heightened competition over natural resources, the need to control market towns, the gradual erosion of social order, and administrative breakdown caused by demographic pressures.[113] Lineage feuds as well as interethnic conflicts (*fenlei xiedou*) prevailed throughout the empire, but were more common in the south-east, where the institution of the lineage had grown more powerful than in the north. The militarisation of powerful lineages reinforced folk models of kinship solidarity, in turn forcing more loosely organised associations to form a unified descent group under the leadership of the gentry. At the level of the court too, ideologies of descent became increasingly important, in particular with the erosion of a sense of cultural identity among Manchu aristocrats. Racial identity through patrilineal descent became important in the Qianlong period (1736–95), when the court progressively turned towards a rigid taxonomy of distinct descent lines (*zu*) to distinguish between Han, Manchu, Mongol and Tibetan.[114] Within three distinct social levels – popular culture, gentry society and court politics – there was widespread invocation of patrilineal descent in the creation and maintenance of group boundaries.

The interest in the control of sexual reproduction culminated in the movement for political reform in the 1890s, which openly sought to challenge imperial institutions and orthodox ideology. The 1898 reformers proposed to

113 H.J. Lamley, 'Hsieh-tou: The pathology of violence in south-eastern China', *Ch'ing-shih Wen-t'i*, 3, no. 7 (Nov. 1977), pp. 1–39.
114 Pamela Kyle Crossley, 'The Qianlong retrospect on the Chinese-martial (*hanjun*) banners', *Late Imperial China*, 10, no. 1 (June 1989), pp. 63–107, and 'Thinking about ethnicity in early modern China', *Late Imperial China*, 11, no. 1 (June 1990), p. 20.

strengthen the country in its confrontation with foreign powers by reforming the thought and behaviour of all the people. They were perhaps the first to articulate a distinctly nationalist agenda of reform in which all citizens would participate in the revival of the country. Moreover, in contrast to their precursors, they promoted an alternative body of knowledge which derived its legitimacy independently of the official examination system. The new knowledge deployed by the reformers was the product of a fusion between different indigenous strains of knowledge and foreign discursive repertoires. An important object of political attention was the species: the scientific category of 'race' and the administrative category of 'population' were heralded as objects worthy of systematic investigation.[115] Modernising reformers like Liang Qichao and Kang Youwei reconfigured lineage discourse into a racial identity which represented all inhabitants of China as the patrilineal descendants of the Yellow Emperor. Extrapolating from an indigenous vision of lineage feuds, which permeated the social landscape of late imperial China, the reformers ordered mankind into a racial hierarchy of biological groups where 'yellows' competed with 'whites' over degenerate breeds of 'browns', 'blacks' and 'reds'. Thriving on its affinity with lineage discourse, 'race' (*huangzhong, zhongzu, renzhong*) gradually emerged as the most common symbol of national cohesion, permanently replacing more conventional emblems of cultural identity. The threat of racial extinction (*miezhong*) – a powerful message of fear based on more popular anxieties about lineage extinction (*miezu*) – was often invoked to bolster the reformers' message of change: 'They will enslave us and hinder the development of our spirit and body. [...] The brown and black races constantly

115 For a much more detailed analysis of the reformers, see Frank Dikötter, chapter 3, 'Race as Lineage', *The discourse of race in modern China*, London: C. Hurst, Stanford University Press, Hong Kong University Press, 1992, pp. 61–96.

waver between life and death: why not the 400 million yellows?'[116]

Correlative to the emergence of a racialised sense of identity, many prominent reformers proclaimed that the wealth and power of the nation were based on the population's physical strength. For instance, Yan Fu (1853–1921) advocated a ban on early marriage, referring to the poor reproduction of the lower strata of society: 'Children feed on coarse food and live in filthy places; they are not properly bred, growing up amid disease and distress: the body becomes weak and the mind turns muddled. When they grow up, lust appears but intelligence stays dormant; they are anxious to take a wife, thereby spreading the wrong seed [zhong, 'race'] from one generation to the next.'[117] Yan Fu, Liang Qichao, Kang Youwei and others in turn emphasised the regulation of human reproduction and the disciplining of individual behaviour for the sake of the nation. One of the first to endow the traditional lore of foetal education with a veil of scientific respectability, Kang Youwei even suggested that superior women should be selected to be impregnated in a Foetal Education Institute (taijiaoyuan) for the propagation of the species. While inferior births would be eliminated by doctors in the Spartan manner so much admired by the reformers (the disabled and the mentally defective would be sterilised), nurses would take care of the delivery, census officers would record new births, and the population office would name the successfully selected infants who would be placed in special institutions.[118] More than ever before, human reproduction appeared as an object

116 Yan Fu, *Yan Fu shiwen xuan* (Selected poems and writings of Yan Fu), Beijing: Renmin wenxue chubanshe, 1959, p. 22.

117 Yan Fu, 'Baozhong yuyi' (Afterthoughts on the preservation of the race) in *Yan Fu ji* (Collected works of Yan Fu), Beijing: Zhonghua shuju, 1986, p. 87.

118 See part 6, chapters 2 and 3 of Kang Youwei, *Datongshu* (One World), Beijing: Guji chubanshe, 1956; partial translation in Laurence G. Thompson, *Ta t'ung shu: The one world philosophy of K'ang Yu-wei*, London: Geo. Allen and Unwin, 1958.

of inquiry, a target of intervention, and the link between individual behaviour and the fortunes of the state. For the 1898 reformers and their successors, the disciplining of individual sexual conduct and the regulation of the population's reproduction had become a significant key to wealth and power. Birth defects and eugenics would become an even greater preoccupation for those modernising élites who embraced 'science' after the fall of the empire in 1911.

3

'DEFECTIVE GENES':
THE REGULATION OF REPRODUCTION
IN REPUBLICAN CHINA

THE MEDICALISATION AND PUBLIC DISPLAY OF
MONSTERS

The imperial reformers failed to secure the power necessary to implement their vision of change. Their critique of the established social order, however, culminated after the fall of the Qing empire in 1911, a momentous political event which was marked by the rapid transformation of the traditional gentry into powerful new élites, such as factory managers, bankers, lawyers, doctors, scientists, educators and journalists. New economic opportunities created through contacts with Western traders and the closer integration of the country into a global economy resulted in the gradual emergence of new social formations, which became especially pronounced in the large metropoles of the coast. The First World War was a period of prosperity for the economy of the coastal regions, which benefited both from the replacement of the imperial system by a republican one and from the decline of European world trade. During this 'golden age' of economic expansion,[1] cities like Tianjin, Nanjing, Shanghai, Wuhan and Canton became the outposts of modernisation. Based on a common ground of social values, a sophisticated network of relations linked intellectuals, urban notables and financial élites together into a modernising avant-garde.

With the collapse of the imperial system, Confucian

---

1 Marie-Claire Bergère, *The golden age of the Chinese bourgeoisie, 1911–1937,* Cambridge University Press, 1989.

knowledge rapidly lost its credibility and authority.[2] Previously imagined as a purposeful whole, a benevolent structure which could not exist independently from ethical forces, 'nature' (*ziran*) was now conceptualised as a set of relatively impersonal forces that could be objectively investigated. No longer were physical bodies thought of as being linked to the cosmological foundations of the universe: bodies were produced according to biological laws inherent to 'nature'. With the decline of conformity to the moral imperatives enshrined in a canon of Confucian texts, a growing number of social thinkers believed 'truth' to be encoded in a nature which only science could decrypt: identity and ancestry were buried deep inside the body. Embryology or genetics, and not philology or paleography, could establish truth. Republican China was characterised by an intense faith in the capacity of 'science' to dismantle 'tradition' and to achieve its opposite, dubbed 'modernity'. 'Science' (*kexue*) became a talisman for universal truth, to be used with a crusading zeal to regenerate culture and society. It was seen as a holistic, unified and monolithic understanding which could provide ultimate truth in all domains.

With the spread of an alternative epistemology based on scientific knowledge, a new medical semiology of the monster appeared, in which the causes of malformation were firmly attributed to purely physical factors. No longer considered to be a heavenly sign, the misshapen creature became an example of medical pathology for the scientist, while hereditary deformities and genetic malformations highlighted the power of natural laws. The language of medical science also made possible a much higher degree of specification, as an indeterminate vocabulary of 'imbalance' and 'deficiency' gave way to a new epistemology of the

---

2 This paragraph draws on some of the conclusions reached in Frank Dikötter, *Sex, culture and modernity in China: Medical science and the construction of sexual identities in the early republican period*, London: Hurst and Honolulu: Hawaii University Press, 1995.

monstrous. Teratology, the 'science of deformed foetuses' (*jitaixue*), discovered new species of monsters, mapped unknown organic disorders, classified pathological cases into modern medical taxonomies, and finally established firmer boundaries between normality and abnormality. The 'monster foetus' (*guaitai*) with 'freakish features' (*jixing guaizhuang*) was represented as being in opposition to the 'normal features' (*zhengchang de xingtai*) of mankind.

As the medical gaze explored hitherto uncharted territories inside the body, hidden defects, interior malformations and organic disorders were brought to light. Medical science not only went increasingly beyond the visible to specify the invisible, which had come to be highlighted thanks to the new tools of anatomy and physiology, but also entered into the realm of potential malformations. Genetics traced the causes of birth defects back to the genes of both parents before conception had even taken place. Increasingly detailed specification of bodily defects inevitably led to much stricter definitions of ill-health. *As a Science of hygiene for women* put it in 1918, 'What is normal and what is healthy are two different things. A human body without structural or functional defects is called normal. Yet some people may have no apparent defects in their internal organs and still be unhealthy, whereas others may have defects which do not directly affect their health, such as an inclined and uneven skull, irregular teeth or malformed ears: these are all called abnormal.'[3]

Freaks occupied a whole new range of discursive spaces, from examples of medical pathology in teratological treatises to illustrations of the dire consequences of poor genetic counselling in popular manuals of marital advice. If official records had taken note of the inauspicious births which were brought to the attention of the emperor before 1911, modern newspapers reported in great detail the appearance of

3 Ge Shaolong, *Nüzi weishengxue* (Science of hygiene for women), Shanghai: Youzheng shuju, 1918, p. 6.

monsters to the general public.[4] Next to photographs of exotic places, distant peoples, famous thinkers and rare species, pictures of monsters appeared in illustrated magazines for the entertainment of the general reader interested in 'natural' phenomena. Scientific knowledge about freaks appeared as a sign of modernity: it demonstrated a commitment to reason, an interest in science and a critical attitude towards more traditional modes of knowledge. Popular teratology partook of a new 'scientific culture' which was specific to the modernising élites of the coastal cities and distinct from what was disparagingly dubbed 'traditional culture'.

The visibility of disfigured people was not only significantly enhanced by the construction of new types of knowledge, but also by their greater prominence in social spaces like fairs and exhibitions. Teratological births were probably offered to the public gaze on fairground stalls throughout the republican period, although references to freak shows are difficult to find in the written record. An infant born with both a vagina and a penis, for instance, caused a stir in the township of Lanbian in 1934, where

4 A few examples taken from newspapers in the mid-1930s include 'Haimen fu chansheng liang guaihai' (A woman from Haimen gives birth to two monster children), *Shenbao*, 4 April 1934, 3:9; 'Songjiang Lu xing fu chansheng guaihai' (Monster child born to Ms Lu in Songjiang), *Shenbao*, 14 July 1934, 3:11; 'Xiaohai you ertou, yitou hanshui, yitou qingxing' (Baby has two heads, one asleep, one awake), *Shenbao*, 23 May 1934, 3:10; 'Nongfu chan guaihai bikong zhong paixie fenzhi' (Peasant girl gives birth to monster child which excretes through nostrils), *Xianggang gongshang*, 13 July 1935, 4:2; 'Mian fu sheng youjiao yinghai' (Woman from Mian gives birth to infant with horns), *Guangmin ribao*, 10 September 1934, 4:1; 'Shiri neng yan zhi guaiying' (Strange infant can speak after ten days), *Xianggang gongshang*, 11 July 1935, p. 3; 'Longchuan chusheng bashiri neng yan guaiying' (Strange infant from Longchuan can speak after eighty days), *Xianggang gongshang*, 17 Sep. 1935, 2:4; 'Meixian Lumou zhi qi yi tai san zi luodi jie neng yan' (Triplets of woman from Mei county all speak at birth), *Xianggang gongshang*, 30 Nov. 1935, 2:4; 'Qiying yangju quan wu shen nang jida' (Strange infant has huge testicles but no kidneys), *Xingzhou ribao*, 6 February 1936, 3:12.

neighbours fought to catch a glimpse of the monster.[5] A year later, a child with two penises was exhibited on fairgrounds in Hong Kong in 1935: his mother charged a few cents for admission but was later arrested for cruelty.[6] Animals with various malformations also went on show, and two-headed snakes and turtles became the key attraction of an exhibit of the Shanghai Daxin Company in 1938.[7] Framed by a photograph or exhibited on a fair, the higher visibility of freaks reflected cultural anxieties over human identity and bodily disintegration: it expressed a need to minimalise angst in times from which certainties were banished. From imperial reports to popular exhibitions, the fascination with the abnormal was localised and domesticated.[8] It was put under a glass-bell, elevated on a pedestal or enshrined in a frame: the material borders of the photograph symbolised the finite categories assigned to that which was different and expressed the social distance from which it could be safely observed.

NATIONALISM, DEGENERATION AND SOFT INHERITANCE IN REPUBLICAN CHINA

A grotesque carnival of freaks and monsters, a macabre procession of sick people, cripples and hunchbacks, a bedraggled humanity crushed under the weight of inbreeding and mental retardation trekked through the pages of medical texts. Malformed infants came to be symbolic representations of

5 'Zhongshanxian Lanbianxu faxian liangxing guaiying' (Infant with two sexes discovered on the market of Lanbian in Zhongshan county), *Gongshang ribao*, 2 June 1934, 2:4.
6 'Qiguai xiaotong liangge shengzhiqi zai Dadadi chenlie' (Monster child with two sexual organs exhibited on the Dada Ground), *Xianggang gongshang*, 30 May 1935, 3:2.
7 Zhu Xi, *Danshengren yu renshengdan* (The evolution of sex), Shanghai: Wenhua shenghuo chubanshe, 1939, p. 141.
8 On the link between representation and confinement, see Sander L. Gilman, *Disease and representation: Images of illness from madness to AIDS*, Ithaca, NY: Cornell University Press, 1988, pp. 19–49.

racial degeneration, while freaks embodied the disfigurement of the nation. Raising the spectre of racial extinction, many writers claimed that the poor physical quality of the population was one of the key causes of the nation's backwardness. The strengthening of the population and the improvement of the race were represented as the essential prerequisites for national survival, an immense effort in which every single individual was meant to participate actively by closely monitoring his or her reproductive potential.[9] New medical vocabularies were thus eagerly embraced by modernising élites in republican China, which enabled them to put increasing stress on the responsibility of both parents in the production of healthy offspring. A clearer delineation of the boundaries of the body and an increased sense of the person became important. The causes of disease were located deeper inside the body, and belief in the relative autonomy of the person gradually spread. Health was said to be determined by the individual's own actions, an approach bolstered by notions of bodily 'resistance' and 'weakness'. Human agency and causality were underlined in a medical discourse which constituted the person as a site of sexual desire and as the essential locus for its proper control: in this period of intense nationalism, the regulation of reproduction became a great concern.

Medical discourse not only constituted individual bodies as crucial sites for the control of sexual desire but also subordinated them to a larger organic collectivity called the 'race' or the 'nation'. Individual self-discipline for the sake of the nation – a modern reconfiguration of the neo-Confucian ideal of self-cultivation – was at the heart of medical discourse in republican China: it stressed the duties of individuals to the collectivity rather than the defence of their rights against the state. Nations, according to the intellectual and political élites, were not merely rational political units, but

9 This aspect of sexual knowledge has been explored in some detail in Dikötter, *Sex, culture and modernity in China*.

organic beings endowed with a unique individuality which should be treasured by all its members: nature and history, rather than mere consent or law, were considered to be the forces binding the individual to the nation. As in Italy and Germany during the same period, the ideal of universal citizenship rights was not very popular; modernising élites insisted that the presumed natural divisions between nations and within the nation be respected.[10]

Just as nations were claimed to be separated by natural divisions, many nationalist writers viewed the members of the nation to be naturally interdependent units rather than merely equal citizens. It considered social hierarchies to have been preordained by nature, since a number of people, notably children, women and 'savages', had not yet evolved through the higher stages of biological development. Social hierarchies were not only seen to be virtually irremediable, since they were imagined to be the result of biological determinants more or less fixed at birth, but also perfectly in accord with natural laws: gender relations, for instance, were thought of as being based on natural sexual distinctions which predestined women to be the passive counterparts to the more active endowments of men; both were joined in an interdependent and complementary union in the same way as the mobile sperm penetrated the nurturing egg to form new life. The appearance of malformations at the bottom of this natural hierarchy could only spell disaster.

This holistic vision of social order, in which individuals were portrayed as self-disciplining cells subordinated to a larger collectivity, was supported by a very flexible approach to biological inheritance. Although a variety of theories on heredity appeared in medical texts, modernising intellectuals in early republican China did not on the whole subscribe to the belief that inheritance was entirely determined by 'genes'. Contrary to the doctrine of genetic determinism,

---

10 For observations on organic nationalism in Europe, see John Hutchinson, *The dynamics of cultural nationalism*, London: Geo. Allen and Unwin, 1987.

according to which all the significant characteristics of a person are firmly inscribed in the genes and cannot be significantly altered, they viewed inheritance as a flexible process which could be improved by human intervention. In what we propose here to call a model of 'soft inheritance', as opposed to the 'hard inheritance' of genetic determinism, the future parents of a child could enhance the quality of their offspring before, during and after conception; this was because inheritance was thought to be a malleable process open to alteration by human agency. While medical theories in late imperial China represented foetal health as a property determined by individual behaviour in conjunction with broader cosmological forces, so too the new medical vocabularies located the laws of inheritance within natural forces which could be favourably inflected by human intervention. A vision of soft inheritance was embedded in the very term 'genetics' (*yichuanxue*), which was not so much a science of genes as a 'science of heredity' in which the material left behind to the next generation remained unspecified.

Contrary to neo-Darwinist theories, which refuted the idea that social advances could be transmitted via genetic inheritance, the theory of the inheritance of acquired characteristics which posited that favourable features acquired in a life-time could be transmitted to the next generation was popular in the 1910s and '20s.[11] The idea that improvements in the environment could lead to genetic changes in the 'race' was part of the neo-Lamarckian paradigm: the close link existing between racial betterment and social progress indicated that every individual should participate in the national effort of modernisation. Neo-Lamarckian theories also viewed evolution as an inevitable ascent through a preordained hierarchy of developmental stages on a ladder. Rejecting the neo-Darwinist explanations of evolution as an

---

11 Differences between neo-Darwinism and neo-Lamarckism in evolutionary theories current in modern China are explored in Dikötter, *The discourse of race*, pp. 97–107.

open-ended process governed by natural selection, adaptation and random mutation, the unilinear model of neo-Lamarckian evolution posited that natural design and universal progress guided the human embryo in a purposeful way through a number of predetermined stages towards maturity. Foetal abnormalities were explained as regressions on the forward march of evolution, as the embryo had failed *in utero* to evolve from a lower stage of organic life towards full humanity. The concept of recapitulation was central to neo-Lamarckian approaches, since embryological growth was imagined to pass through the earlier stages of evolution, starting with the amoeba and ascending to the level of fish, reptile and finally mammal. Within this symbolic universe, monsters became the ominous signs of racial degeneration, the portents of national decline, the embodiment of a failure to harness the natural forces of progress. Theories of degeneration were the reverse side of a strong belief in unilinear evolution, in which time was articulated as an axis with one direction only: forwards. *Jinhua*, or 'evolution', meant 'transformation forwards', whereas its antipode *tuihua*, or 'devolution', meant 'transformation backwards'. Devolution stood face to face with evolution, as the race was said to be in a crucial phase of change in which biological degeneration was a natural retribution for social decay.

If biologising metaphors of the nation as a sick person prevailed and a focus upon procreation and maternity became widespread, ideological differences and contradictory conclusions also marked the field of medical science. Incompatible theories were invoked, contradictory ideas were bandied around, and vague phrases on 'struggle for survival' were widespread. Overlapping biological myths and conflicting notions of evolution formed a common repertoire which was sometimes used in the most arbitrary way by authors who regarded themselves as progressive. In the confused invocation of biological ideas, social thinkers, medical writers and liberal intellectuals disagreed over the relative importance of nurture versus nature. Contrary to the more popular theories of neo-Lamarckism, for instance, Mendelian laws also started to circulate in both learned and popular literature from the mid-1920s onwards to show how genetic factors determined the endowment of an individual at birth. As genetics became a more widespread field in the 1930s, some experts in the field of human biology (Chen Jianshan, Chen Zhen, Wang Qishu) even started systematically to challenge the theory of acquired characteristics.[12] Generally, however, the model of soft inheritance proposed a more flexible vision in which nature and nurture were seen as mutually interdependent factors in a child's heredity. This model established a strong connection between individual health and national well-being. In a representation of society as an organism for which regenerating therapies should be prescribed, human beings were said to have a responsibility for the health of the seedling at every stage of the reproductive process. 'Poor' characteristics were seen not so much as being cast in the iron language of genes but as being gradually acquired during conception and pregnancy. The seed, the womb, even childhood and adolescence imparted influences upon a person that were all thought to be part of 'heredity'. Nefarious influences could turn a healthy body into a sickly monster at virtually every stage of organic growth.

This is not to say that 'genes' were considered as being relatively insignificant elements in this particular model of inheritance. On the contrary, because 'genes' were represented as flexible entities open to change over time, they were endowed with enormous powers which had to be carefully monitored by every individual. 'Genes' (*jiyin*) were literally 'fundamental factors' (*jiben yinsu*) in human heredity. A strong belief in somatisation entailed that virtually every mental, moral or social characteristic of a person could be

12 See for instance Chen Jianshan, *Taijiao* (Foetal education), Shanghai: Shangwu yinshuguan, 1926, Chen Zhen, *Putong shengwuxue* (General biology), Shanghai: Shangwu yinshuguan, 1924, Wang Qishu, *Yichuanxue gailun* (Introduction to heredity), Shanghai: Shangwu yinshuguan, 1926.

seen to have a genetic basis that was transmitted to the next generation via sexual intercourse. Adequate restraint and strict selection were necessary before engaging in the act of reproduction: if eugenics prescribed a ban on reproduction for categories of people judged to be socially and biologically deviant – from criminals and alcoholics to the mad and the bad – every person harboured potentially harmful features which might imperil future offspring. Reiterating an old taboo under the guise of medical science, it was claimed that drinking before sexual intercourse could lead to disabled descendants, since it destroyed the spermatozoa transmitted during the act. The genetic capital of each individual was thus inexorably linked to the gene pool of the nation.

'THE INTERMEDIATE SEX':
EMBRYOLOGY, HERMAPHRODITISM
AND GENDER DISTINCTIONS

Detailed scientific studies of congenital malformations were published in republican China. Their purpose, however, was not to discover new knowledge in an inductive effort to construct better hypotheses, but to demonstrate the power of science to throw light on all aspects of life. 'Science' became a holistic philosophy of absolute truth which tolerated no alternative explanations. Social reformers undertook to educate the nation about human anatomy and embryology under the banner of science. Reflecting the cultural withdrawal of learned literature from folk culture, social reformers dedicated to the education of the general public decried popular errors about hermaphroditism. Their admonitions against 'superstition' (*mixin*) were couched in learned treatises on popular errors, a genre not dissimilar to Laurent Joubert's *Erreurs populaires au fait de la médecine* of the sixteenth century. Liu Piji, to take one such example, inveighed against popular misconceptions about sex transformations and highlighted instead the physiology of hermaphrodites: 'With fake hermaphrodites, it happens that the male changes into a female and the female changes into a male. His inner physiology may be without any defect, but the outer part is not completely formed. It happens that the body undergoes many changes at puberty and that the outer part fully develops and reveals itself in its true appearance. There have been cases like this throughout history. Traditionally, people did not understand the reasons for these changes and called fake hermaphrodites "sex transformation demons". It is a common phenomenon which official histories and popular gazetteers have recorded as an inauspicious sign. In reality, it is nothing but a very ordinary phenomenon; what is there to be surprised about?'[13] Within medical discourse, the hermaphrodite was thus transformed from a deviant creature to a perfectly normal example of mankind's androgynous nature.

Embryological knowledge in particular was mobilised to demonstrate that male and female bodies evolved from a common foetal stage. Many textbooks on embryology in republican China underlined that in the male embryo the female features gradually atrophied and degenerated, whereas in the female embryo the outer male organ disappeared. The emphasis on a shared embryological development even led to a number of writers claiming that the male foetus was also initially endowed with breasts. A sign of arrested development, they were thought to have 'degenerated' (tuihua) during the last month in the womb, as the foetus evolved towards a higher stage. Much as the human foetus had evolved out of an ape-like embryo, the male transcended the female in the last stage of growth – so wrote Chen Yucang in his popular *Life and physiology*.[14] In line with the theory of recapitulation, which held that embryological growth passed through the earlier stages of evolution, the female was pic-

13 Liu Piji, *Renjian wujie de shengwu* (Misinterpretations in everyday biology), Shanghai: Shangwu yinshuguan, 1928, p. 95.
14 Chen Yucang, *Shenghuo yu shengli* (Life and physiology), Taipei: Zhengzhong shuju, 1958, pp. 208–9.

tured as a vessel of evolutionary traits which had been transcended by the male. The repository of a lost phylogeny, woman was a man not fully evolved. Hermaphrodites, within this vision of gender distinctions, were interpreted as intermediate types: 'However, it happens that the sexual organs of both sexes appear together on one body: these people are generally called *yin* and *yang* people [*yinyangren*].' This was the view of gynaecologist Gui Zhiliang, who classified hermaphrodites into 'real half *yin* half *yang*' (*zhenxing ban yinyang*) and 'fake half *yin* half *yang*' (*jiaxing ban yinyang*), explaining that only the former had completely formed testicles and ovaries.[15] While the dwarfed penis resembled a small clitoris in the male hermaphrodite, the female counterpart was represented as a stout and hairy being who concealed a womb under a masculine appearance: both were paraded as intermediate products of male and female bodies.

Even as new medical sciences like embryology and comparative anatomy enabled modernising intellectuals to locate the mechanisms of sex differentiation inside the human body, a more holistic vision continued to emphasise the importance of the environment. Sex transformations could be induced by a change in the environment, as some medical reports were keen to demonstrate: in one case, a young man who breast-fed his child after the death of his wife developed mammary glands. Reminiscent of older theories in which bodily fluids could transform themselves into sweat, semen or milk, it seemed that the hormones circulating in the blood could be directly influenced by environmental changes.[16] Outside medical circles, popular stories about sex transformations – based on a holistic vision in which the social and the biological were closely interrelated – regularly appeared in the daily press, such as the case of Wang Lin, who had

15 Gui Zhiliang, *Nüren zhi yisheng* (A woman's life), Peking: Zhengzhong shuju, 1936, p. 11.
16 Zhu Zhenjiang, *Rufang ji qita* (About breasts and other things), Shanghai: Kaiming shudian, 1933, p. 102.

'caused a sensation throughout town' (*hongdong quanshi*): at the age of eighteen, his penis receded, his face became smooth, he lacked physical strength, was rapidly exhausted and 'behaved like a girl', until he was found to be two months pregnant after having developed an intimate relationship with a neighbour.[17] Such stories raised the frightful possibility that social deviance could entail a biological transformation: a man could well become a woman by behaving like one.[18]

Popular neo-Lamarckian theories, which represented women as a lower stage on the evolutionary ladder, were endorsed by more elaborate investigations into the nature of hermaphroditism. Zhu Xi (1900–62), a professor at Sun Yatsen University in Canton and an authority in the field of reproductive biology, carefully analysed the sexual organs of a number of hermaphrodites which he classified as the 'intermediate sex' of the human species: in a reconfiguration of older notions of gender hierarchy, the female hermaphrodite was seen as the 'lower level of the intermediate sex', the male counterpart was renamed the 'higher level of the intermediate sex'.[19] Since women were a grade below men on the evolutionary ladder, female hermaphrodites were said to be more common, as evolutionary forces always strove forwards.

17 This story was reported as 'Junshao nan'er bian shaonü' (A handsome boy changes into a young girl), *Gongshang ribao*, 1 May 1934, 4:3.

18 For similar stories, see 'Yinyangren' (Hermaphrodism), *Shenbao*, 25 February 1935, 4:16; 'Nü hua nan zhi kaozheng' (Research into transformations of female into male), *Xinwenbao*, 20 March 1935, 4:14; Fan Shoujian, 'Nü bian nan shen de tantao' (Inquiry into transformations of female into male), *Beiping chenbao*, 21 March 1935, p. 8; 'Nü hua nan shen kexueshang de jieshi' (Scientific explanation for transformations of female into male), *Xinwenbao*, 19 August 1935, 4:13; 'Nanxing bian nüxing de shiyan' (Experiments in transformations of male into female), 16 December 1935, *Xinwenbao*, 4:113; 'Neifenmi de ezuo — nan bian nü yu nü bian nan' (The evil function of hormones and sex transformations), *Xianggang gongshang*, 2 September 1936, p. 7.

19 Zhu Xi, *Cixiong zhi bian* (The changes of female and male), Shanghai: Wenhua shenghuo chubanshe, 1945, pp. 309–12.

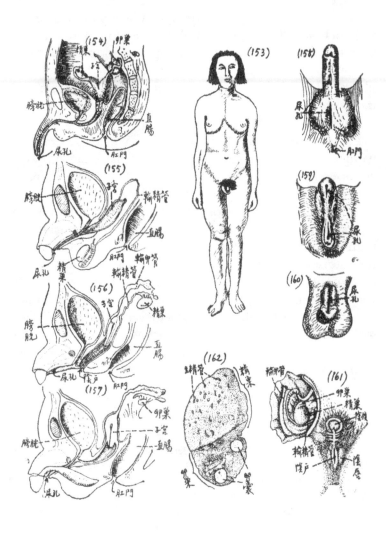

The development of hermaphroditism.

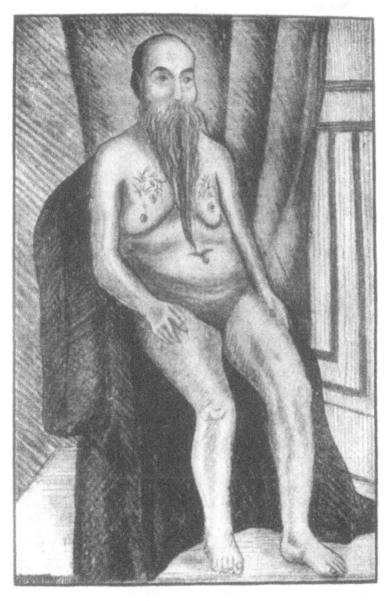

Madeleine Lefort, an eighteenth-century French hermaphrodite.

The importance Zhu Xi gave to hermaphrodites in his discussion of gender distinctions – thought to be biologically determined structures – was evident in his choice of an illustration of a female hermaphrodite, placed just after the title page of his book entitled *The changes of female and male* (1945). The picture showed a bearded women with a hairy chest and a long beard, its impact on the reader enhanced by her reflective appearance and a mandarinal posture (a straight back, both hands on the lap and the legs evenly spread). This illustration represented Marie-Madeleine Lefort, a bearded lady who had presented herself at the public Hôtel-Dieu in Paris in 1864 for treatment of chronic pleurisy.[20] She was autopsied after her death in hospital two months later: half a century later, she had become a cultural icon of the androgynous nature of the human species on the other side of the world.

Scientific notions of gender in republican China revealed profound ambiguities about the nature of masculinity and femininity, and many writers explored hermaphroditism to highlight the basic kinship between man and woman. In contrast to the views of some medical writers in England, France and Germany, women were rarely thought of as being a different species with incommensurably different organs and functions.[21] Rather than representing women as equal but different individuals of a pluralistic society, medical dis-

20 For the original picture, see the lowbrow book by Martin Howard, *Victorian grotesque: An illustrated excursion into medical curiosities, freaks and abnormalities, principally of the Victorian age*, London: Jupiter, 1977, p. 39.

21 Thomas W. Laqueur, *Making sex: Body and gender from the Greeks to Freud*, Cambridge, MA: Harvard University Press, 1990. This book's thesis of a radical vision of male and female incommensurability elaborated by male authors to oppose liberal claims in favour of sexual equality, however, might need some qualification. Hermaphroditism, as a symbol of a basic kinship between men and women, was not only important in legal and medical debates in the eighteenth century (Jacques Marx, 'Descriptions géographiques et mythiques au XVIIe siècle', *Revue Roumaine d'Histoire*, 22, no. 4 (1983), pp. 357–69; Andrea Gloria Michler, 'Ambiguità e transmutazione. Discussioni mediche e giuridiche in epoca moderna (secoli XVII e XVIII)', *Memoria i Revista di Storia delle Donne*, no. 24 (1988), pp. 43–60), but remained an important theme even in late nineteenth

course tended to think of men and women as complementary beings who formed interdependent parts of an organic collectivity.[22] Biologising discourses of the body in republican China reflected a tension between the idea of gender hierarchy, in which female bodies were the passive counterparts of active male bodies, and a vision of modernity in which men and women were undifferentiated members of an organic collectivity. As in the late imperial period, hermaphroditism remained a symbol of the ambivalent nature of human sexuality and demonstrated the fundamental kinship of men and women. 'Monsters', in other words, remained epiphenomena of a holistic world order. Scientific investigations into human malformations remained illustrative rather than deductive, and few analogical forms of construction were made between evidence and theory.

TERATOLOGY, RECAPITULATION AND HEREDITY

'Freaks' were rarely discussed as full human beings in their own right anywhere in the modern world. Medical discourse

century Europe. The feminisation of the male, the masculinisation of the female and androgyny as the image of a quintessential humanity were not uncommon in medical science as well as in artistic circles, particularly in Art Nouveau and Dadaism (Christina von Braun, 'Männliche Hysterie, Weibliche Askese: Zum Paradigmenwechsel in den Geschlechterrollen' in Karin Rick (ed.), *Das Sexuelle, die Frauen und die Kunst*, Tübingen, pp. 10ff, no date). The idea of male menstruation was important in the medical literature of nineteenth-century Europe, an expression of the fascination with the problem of hermaphroditism as a sign of human bisexuality (Ornella Moscucci, 'Hermaphroditism and sex difference: The construction of gender in Victorian England' in Marina Benjamin (ed.), *Science and sensibility: Gender and scientific enquiry, 1780–1945*, London: Blackwell, 1991, pp. 174–99).

22 When Margaret Sanger visited China in 1922, Hu Shi and a number of businessmen and professional people discussed with her the possibility of creating a neuter gender such as the workers in a beehive or an ant-hill; see Margaret Sanger, *An autobiography*, New York: Dover Publications, 1971, p. 342.

defined children with congenital malformations as pathological cases to be eliminated rather than as potential persons
with disabilities to be lived with. More important, tributary
of the retributive tradition, medical discourse in China often
confused causality with finality: 'monsters' were used to illustrate broader social issues beyond the individual cases
described. Much as birth defects were brandished to highlight the responsibilities of both parents in the production of
eugenic offspring, hermaphrodites were used to debate the
nature of gender distinctions. In popular culture, the persistence of customary beliefs in wonders and marvels was most
visible in newspapers, where freaks such as the child who
could speak in its mother's womb continued to enchant the
less educated sectors of the public. One Hong Kong daily
brought the case of a woman who had been pregnant for
three years to the attention of the public. Her triplets imparted a message of peace at the moment of birth: the first infant
said 'This year peace will spread', the second 'Next year
peace will extend', and the third 'The year after next the
people will find peace'; the wondrous trio then immediately
expired.[23] The news item which reported such cases
enshrined the abnormal and assigned it a place within an
established cosmology. On the borders of reality, liminal
figures allowed popular writers to explore regions of ambiguity and turn reason on its head. The news item about
monsters played on the attraction of the irrational: it became
a privileged moment of controlled anxiety in which fears
could be exorcised. As well as being a break through the
monotony of ordered existence, it also created the illusion of
a different universe which lay behind the routine of daily life.

23 'Shiri neng yan zhi guaiying' (Strange infant can speak after ten days),
Xianggang gongshang, 11 July 1935, p. 3; 'Longchuan chusheng bashiri neng yan
guaiying' (Strange infant from Longchuan can speak after eigthy days), *Xianggang
gongshang*, 17 September 1935, 2:4; 'Meixian Lumou zhi qi yi tai san zi luodi jie
neng yan' (Triplets of woman from Mei county all speak at birth), *Xianggang gongshang*, 30 November 1935, 2:4.

Similarly, teratological cases in medical discourse were rarely thought to have any intrinsic human interest in themselves but were merely meant to exemplify broader cultural concerns. New classificatory systems constructed by scientific discourse introduced order and meaning into the random manifestations of nature. Similar to the invention of gender boundaries, in which the hermaphrodite was seen as a sort of hybrid, scientific taxonomies imposed a principle of discontinuity into a realm of continuous variation. Zones of overlap, of continuity or of ambiguity were discarded by medical science in favour of clear-cut boundaries. Categories such as 'genus', 'species' or 'sub-species' were carved out of an indeterminate mosaic as science identified, classified and ranked: if the freak used to be a symbol of radical otherness, an irregularity beyond the reach of the norm, science introduced into the monster an element of intelligibility. Teratology, the scientific investigation of monstrosities, discovered patterns of regularity in the monster, posited as mediator between the normal and the abnormal.[24]

The theory of recapitulation was increasingly invoked to portray the monster as a leap back in time. Previously unconnected malformations were linked through a new explanatory framework which carefully placed monsters on an integrated evolutionary scale. Although the French anthropologist Paul Topinard's standard definition of birth defects was almost half a century old by the 1930s and no longer current in Europe,[25] many medical writers in China would have embraced it: 'Harelip, polydactylia, microcephalia, are, as it were, hesitations of the principles of evolution, attempts on its part to stop at points where it had rested in anterior forms,

24 On the invention of the hybrid, see Jacqueline Duvernay-Bolens, 'Un trickster chez les naturalistes. La notion d'hybride', *Ethnologie Française*, 23, no. 1 (Jan.-March 1993), pp. 142–52.
25 See Stephen Jay Gould, *Ontogeny and phylogeny*, Cambridge, MA: Harvard University Press, 1977, pp. 49–52.

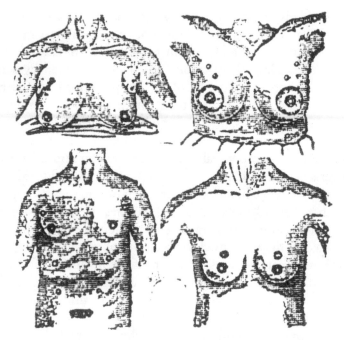

Double pair of breasts.

or to progress in other previously-followed directions.'[26] Monstrous atavisms indicated how easily progress could be inverted to draw mankind back into darkness. Terms like arrested development, vestigial structure, convergent variation and regression were all explained in detail to the reader interested in the power of evolution.[27] Specific cases were brought to the attention of the public: Zhang Zuoren, professor of zoology at Sun Yatsen University, paraded Xue Banghua, a schoolboy aged seven who had four breasts.[28]

26 Cynthia E. Russett, *Sexual science: The Victorian construction of womanhood*, Cambridge, MA: Harvard University Press, 1989, pp. 68–9.

27 For instance, Chen Jianshan, *Taijiao* (Foetal education), Shanghai: Shangwu yinshuguan, 1926, p. 44.

28 Zhang Zuoren, *Renlei tianyan shi* (History of human evolution), Shanghai: Shangwu yinshuguan, 1930, p. 53.

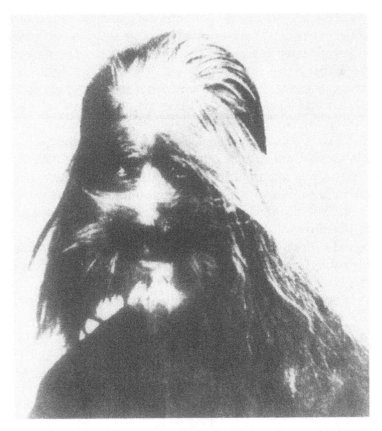

Hairy man Li Baoshu, put on display in Beijing during the 1920s.

Chen Yucang (1889–1947), a foreign-educated doctor who became director of the provincial hospital of Hubei province, director of the Medical College of Tongji University and a secretary to the Legislative Yuan, even suspected that mankind's mammal origins lurked behind such bizarre occurrences: if most people had one pair of breasts, evolutionary forces could always add an extra couple of sterile nipples.[29]

29 Chen Yucang, *Shenghuo yu shengli* (Life and physiology), Taipei: Zhengzhong shuju, 1958, p. 209.

Excessive body hair in particular was endowed with evolutionary meaning.[30] As embryological growth was imagined to pass through the earlier stages of evolution, starting with the amoeba and ascending to the level of fish, reptile and finally mammal, the human foetus was thought gradually to lose its hair (called lanugo) after the first seven months. During the late nineteenth century, hypertrichosis, as aberrant hair growth was called, inspired a mass of literature in Europe that was entirely out of proportion to the number of actual cases reported.[31] Scientists devised different taxonomies to impose structure and meaning upon the variety of growth disorders that had been observed.[32] 'Hypertrichosis universalis' or 'hypertrichosis lanuginosa' was considered the most extreme case of aberrant hair growth, in which the patient's face and body were covered with a thick coat of long soft hair: called 'dog-men' or 'ape-men', such cases of extreme hypertrichosis were exhibited for amusement up till the end of the Second World War. Rudolph Virchow in 1873 was the first natural scientist to suggest that aberrant hair growth was a form of arrested development: the persistence of embryonic conditions in the lanugo was thought to be associated with the normal development of the rest of the organism.[33] It was believed to be an atavistic manifestation of

30 On hair as a symbol for gender boundaries, see Frank Dikötter, 'Hairy barbarians, furry primates and wild men: Medical science and cultural representations of hair in China' in Alf Hiltebeitel and Barbara Miller (eds), *Hair in Asian cultures: Context and change*, Albany: State University of New York Press, 1998, pp. 51–74.

31 For instance Arie Geyl, *Beobachtungen und Ideen über Hypertrichose*, Hamburg: Dermatologische Studien, 1890; see also A.E. Cockayne, *Inherited abnormalities of the skin and its appendages*, Oxford University Press, 1933, p. 245.

32 In particular Max Bartels, 'Über abnorme Behaarung beim Menschen', *Zeitschrift für Ethnologie*, 8 (1876), pp. 110–29; Hans Chiari, 'Über Hypertrichosis des Menschen', *Prager Medizinische Wochenschrift*, 15 (1890), pp. 495–7 and 512–15.

33 Rudolph Virchow, 'Die russischen Haarmenschen', *Berliner Klinische Wochenschrift*, 10 (1873), pp. 337–9; for a medical discussion, see Attilio Zanca, 'In tema di hypertrichosis universalis congenita: Contributo storico-medico', *Physis*, 25, no. 1 (1983), pp. 41–66.

the original hairiness of mankind, the reincarnation of man's primitive ancestry. The idea of racial reversion was favourably received by some researchers, but came increasingly under attack during the 1920s and '30s.[34] In China, where neo-Lamarckism had gained considerable currency, the myth of arrested development established a more powerful foothold. Zhang Zuoren reprinted a photograph of a hirsute man 'born in Russia' in his book on the history of human evolution. The picture probably represented Stephen Bilgraski, alias 'Lionel the lion-man', an artist who appeared in freak-shows for many years with Barnum and Bailey at the beginning of the twentieth century.[35] Chinese examples were also provided: in 1921, a certain Miss Wang had given birth to a hairy baby, later exhibited in the Agricultural Experimental Ground of Beijing.[36] The same year, photographs of Chinese 'hairy man' Li Baoshu were put on display in the capital's zoo.[37] The obsession with hair was echoed in the popular press: in an age spellbound by the implications of evolution, reports about 'monsters' covered with hair appeared regularly for the amazement of the public.[38] As in modern Europe, freaks had an appeal which was shared by different levels of

34 C.H. Danforth, *Hair: With special reference to hypertrichosis*, Chicago: American Medical Association, 1925; see also A. Savill, *The hair and the scalp: A clinical study with a chapter on hirsuties*, London: Edward Arnold, 1935.

35 Compare the picture with Daniel P. Mannix, *Freaks: We who are not as others. With rare and amazing photos from the author's personal scrapbook*, San Francisco: Research Publications, 1990, p. 87.

36 Zhang Zuoren, *Renlei tianyan shi* (History of human evolution), Shanghai: Shangwu yinshuguan, 1930, pp. 51–2.

37 The case of Li Baoshu from Hebei province was investigated by anthropologist Liu Xian of Fudan University in Shanghai, although I have been unable to locate the published results of his work.

38 For instance 'Jinghainong chan guai'er bianti sheng baimao' (Monster child covered with white hair born in village of Jinghai), *Xianggang gongshang*, 8 November 1934; 'Kuangzhong mou shouliu bianti changmao guai xiaohai' (Small monster child covered with long hair found in Kuangzhong), *Shenbao*, 20 September 1935.

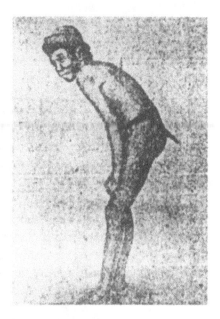

African with a tail.

society.[39] Racial atavism highlighted the fragile nature of the boundary between human and animal: furry beasts were always lurking behind the thin veil of civilisation. You Jiade's *Origins of mankind* (1929), like many other books on human biology in the 1920s and '30s, drew extensively on the theory of recapitulation. The 'fine and long hair' covering the foetus was compared to that of a monkey and was thought to fall out at the moment of birth.[40]

Further proof of man's descent from the monkey was thought to reside in his atrophied tail. If the human was no more than an evolved anthropoid, the 'sons of the Yellow Emperor' (*huangdi zisun*) were merely the 'descendants of apes' (*yuanhou zisun*). The ancestors of the sage Confucius

39 Robert Bogdan, *Freak show: Presenting human oddities for amusement and profit*, University of Chicago Press, 1988.
40 You Jiade, *Renlei qiyuan* (Origins of mankind), Shanghai: Shijie shuju, 1929, p. 7.

had lived in trees, clung to branches with their tails, eating raw meat and drinking blood, with no clothes to protect them from the elements. 'Most people do not wish to hear that man has a tail. But if we dissect the human body we will immediately find proof of the existence of a tail, which consists of three, four or even five coccyxal vertebrae merged together in the lower part of the spine. The human foetus has a tail which is longer than a limb and also has a muscle to wag it. In the grown-up person this muscle survives in the form of a filamentous joint.'[41] In Germany, Liu Piji even reported in his *Misinterpretations in everyday biology*, a boy had been born with a tail 30 centimetres long: 'This is clear proof that civilised people also have a tail!'[42] 'Inferior races', however, were said to be much closer to primitive man, and Africans were sometimes considered to have hairy tails. Periodicals reported newly-discovered 'races' with tails,[43] and titles such as 'Apes have tail; man has tail too' appeared in daily newspapers;[44] reversions of man to ape were also reported.[45]

Evolutionary reversions to an ancestral state were thought to explain the harelip, while the earlobe was represented as a vestigial structure. Mendelian laws of inheritance, however, were also used to account for a number of congenital malformations. Neo-Darwinian explanations based on genetic determinism were either embraced (England and Germany) or resolutely rejected in favour of a more flexible model of

41 Zhang Ziping, *Renlei jinhualun* (The theory of human evolution), Shanghai: Shangwu yinshuguan, 1930, p. 46.
42 Liu Piji, *Renjian wujie de shengwu* (Misinterpretations in everyday biology), Shanghai: Shangwu yinshuguan, 1928, p. 80.
43 'You wei renzhong yu shiren renzhong de faxian' (Discovery of a race of men with tails and a race of cannibals), *Dongfang zazhi*, 26, no. 5 (March 1929), pp. 99–101.
44 'Houzi you weiba renlei ye you weiba' (Apes have tail; man has tail too), *Dagongbao*, 9 January 1936; 'Sheng yi liangzhou zhi daiwei nühai' (Girl with tail already two weeks old), *Zhongyang ribao*, 29 April 1936.
45 'Ren bian hou zhi qiwen' (Strange news about a man changing into an ape), *Beiping chenbao*, 6 June 1935.

neo-Lamarckism (France), but the two approaches were not
seen to be mutually incompatible in a model of soft inheritance which stressed the ability of genes to change over short
periods of time. Genetic knowledge became particularly
popular in the 1930s. Bodily imperfections were used to
illustrate new laws of inheritance: baldness, previously
explained as a deficiency of the kidney, was given in the
1910s as an example of a hereditary defect.[46] Albinism, sometimes seen as a retribution for sexual intercourse during menstruation, was explained by the laws of inheritance. Chen
Yucang considered how 'albinos not only lack pigments in
their skin, but their hair is also white, the eyes are often of a
blue-ash colour or remain colourless; since they are not protected by pigments, albinos cannot resist strong sunrays and
their sight is weak. The yellow race, the white race and the
black race all have albinos; even mammals like cats, dogs, rabbits and rats have albinos. When an albino marries a normal
person, the first generation is not albino, but when the second generation intermarries, according to Mendelian laws,
there is separated inheritance.'[47] On the other hand, the self-
proclaimed scientist Liu Piji, indefatigable destroyer of popular errors, authoritatively invoked the concept of
'degenerative mutation' (tuihua tubian) to throw light on the
genetics of albinism.[48] Elsewhere, Liu Piji's uneven grasp of
the different theories of inheritance became even clearer, as
he happily mixed the theory of acquired characteristics with
genetic laws. Appealing to teratogenic experiments in his
discussion of polydactylia, he argued that chemicals which
were artificially added to the embryo could induce different
congenital malformations. Reminiscent of older notions of
'strength' and 'heat', he explained the appearance of super-

46 Yancheng, 'Fatu zhi yuanyin ji qi yufang' (The reasons and prevention of baldness), Dongfang zazhi, 16, no. 2 (Feb. 1919), pp. 201–2.
47 Chen, Shenghuo, p. 224.
48 Liu Piji, Renjian wujie de shengwu (Misinterpretations in everyday biology),
Shanghai: Shangwu yinshuguan, 1928, p. 102.

numerary fingers as an inherent 'weakness' of the embryo which was compressed by the amnion. These defects, once induced by amniotic compression, could then become hereditary.[49] Other popular writers also continued to adhere to neo-Lamarckian theories while parading a fashionable terminology of 'genes' (*jiyin*) and 'chromosomes' (*ranseti*). The well-intentioned *Advice on childbirth* (1933), meant for the general reader, explained monsters either as a reversion to ancestral features (*fanben yichuan*), highlighting the power of evolution as atavistic features suddenly reappeared in the offspring of a corrupt lineage, or as unhealthy foetal development, endowing parents with a responsibility for foetal health. The author believed that the appearance of superfluous fingers was due to a chromosome which contained an ancestral feature capable of 'suddenly' developing: as mankind had originally evolved from animals, bestial features could resurface from this distant heritage, even leading to monsters with a horn on their head.[50]

Even more directly indebted to older notions of conception, some medical writers distinguished between 'internal factors', such as the quality of the seed, and 'external factors', such as contamination, in the causality of congenital malformations. Ding Shu'an and Zhou Efen's textbook on obstetrics, entitled *Easy obstetrics* (1948), isolated the 'poor quality of the semen' and other unspecified 'hereditary' factors as the main internal causes for the appearance of malformations, while uterine and amniotic diseases as well as chemical or bacterial contamination were seen as external causes: male semen was somehow considered to be the determining factor in conception, while the womb was by implication represented as no more than a convenient receptacle. Both authors boldly established a new taxonomy of monstrous births: 'We

49 Liu Piji, *Shengwu nanti jieda* (Explanations of difficult problems in biology), Shanghai: Shangwu yinshuguan, 1935, p. 12.
50 Wang Yang, *Shengyu guwen* (Advice on childbirth), Shanghai: Zhongyang shuju, 1933, pp. 25–6.

distinguish between single monsters and attached monsters. Single monsters can be further classified into three types: (1) those who lack an organ; (2) those who have a malformed or a misplaced organ; (3) those who have a duplicated or expanded organ. Conjoined monsters are a type of monozygotic twins. The two foetuses have not clearly separated during their development so that they are partly attached and turn into different kinds of monsters. There are symmetrical and asymmetrical twin monsters. Symmetrical monsters can further be divided into the following types: (1) those attached by the back; they have two heads and intact limbs; (2) those with two malformed heads, they have four arms and two legs; (3) those with one head or with both heads attached, they have four arms and four legs. The location where both bodies are linked can vary, hence the many existing differences. Parturition is generally difficult and rarely successful. Both parts should be separated and taken out by embryotomy.'[51] Ranking and classifying was somehow thought by the authors to be an intellectual exercise which had sufficient explanatory power in itself.

If legions were eager to speak in the voice of authority provided by 'science', only a handful actually bothered to base their statements on empirical evidence. In the field of teratology, experimental embryology prevailed in Europe from the late nineteenth century onwards, and publications on malformations and case histories appeared in medical journals. Through interference with the embryo by way of external pressure, chemical contamination or even irradiation, embryologists attempted to verify their hypotheses on the formation of malformations by producing monsters in their own laboratories.[52] Zhu Xi was one of the very few scientists in China

51 Ding Shu'an and Zhou Efen, *Jianyi chankexue* (Easy obstetrics), Beijing: Cicheng yinshuachang, 1948, pp. 194–5.
52 For an introduction, see Jean-Louis Fischer, 'Hérédité et tératologie, 1860–1920' in Claude Bénichou (ed.), *L'ordre des charactères. Aspects de l'hérédité dans l'histoire des sciences de l'homme*, Paris: Vrin, 1989, pp. 95–118.

who participated in the exploration of such new avenues for research. An embryologist of international reputation, he published the most detailed study of teratology in republican China, accompanied by copious hand drawings of micro-cephalia, macrocephalia, cyclopism, polydactylia and other congenital malformations.[53] He explained teratology as a complementary field to embryology, since pathological deviations could illustrate the underlying norm. He stressed the potentialities of the embryo, represented not as a complete creature which simply matured inside the uterus but as a potential being which unfolded in interaction with the uterine milieu. Zhu Xi even discerned 'organ-shaping substances' (*qiguan xingchengzhi*) that activated and controlled the shape of the embryo: malformations were interpreted as the result of damage incurred by these substances via excessive heat, chemicals or lesions. A professor at Sun Yatsen University in Canton and a specialist in the field of artificial parthenogenesis in Chinese frogs, Zhu himself had accidentally induced a teratogenic change in his laboratory experiments with a centrifugal apparatus on frog embryos. His repeated experiments on non-fertilised eggs later in Beijing, which produced a series of freakish frogs with deformed mouths, three eyes or missing limbs, confirmed that a variety of malformations could be artificially induced even before an embryo had taken shape. In a summary published in a learned journal in France, the author hypothesised that the substances which gave shape to different organs had a specific location inside the egg: these substances had been disturbed and displaced by external centrifugal forces and had resulted in the appearance of monstrous frogs.[54]

---

53 Zhu Xi, *Danshengren yu renshengdan* (The evolution of sex), Shanghai: Wenhua shenghuo chubanshe, 1939, p. 141.

54 Tchou-Su, 'Embryons doubles obtenus par la centrifugation des oeufs d'anoures récemment fécondés. Origine des localisations germinales', *Comptes Rendus de la Société de Biologie*, 122 (1936), p. 43; see also Zhu Xi, 'Shiyan de walei shuangtai' (Teratogenic joined frog foetuses), *Shengwuxue zazhi*, 1, no. 3 (1936).

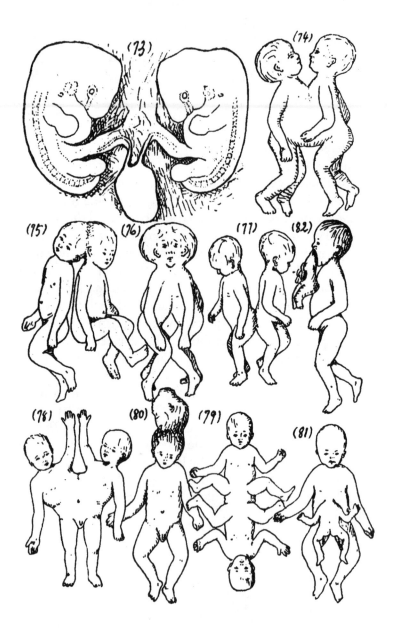

A vision of conjoined twins.

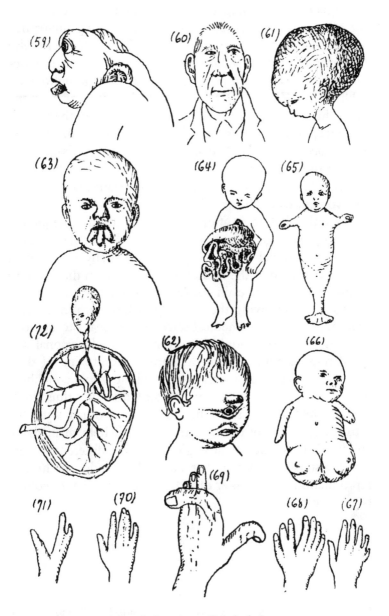

A hand-drawing of birth defects.

Zhu Xi used his experiments to add weight to the theory of epigenesis, according to which organic structures grew out of undifferentiated forms rather than being preformed entities inherent in egg or sperm. His experiments also demonstrated the advantage of treating women as interdependent members in a modernising nation: throughout his publications, Zhu Xi always took up the cause of women's rights, highlighting the importance of women in the process of conception and reproduction (in another book entitled *Women over men*, published in 1941, he even envisaged that women might one day procreate without men).[55] The implication of his experiments on frogs' eggs meant that the ovum of a woman, when disturbed by external pressure or a sudden shock, either before or after fertilisation, could subsequently develop grave organic malformations. Rather than displacing a more traditional vision of gender hierarchy which kept women confined to the household, his study on the contrary assigned women an even greater responsibility over reproduction by identifying the womb as a biological marker. If anatomy was destiny, medical science was meant to demonstrate that women should be given increased personal and social responsibilities, since the careful monitoring of their bodies and regulated procreative behaviour would contribute healthy offspring to the nation. Medical discourse thus closely associated the personal health of the woman with the future well-being of the nation. From self-help manuals on childbirth to learned teratological treatises, different discursive registers all stressed that better knowledge of human reproduction was a matter of individual as much as of collective interest.

55 Zhu Xi, *Zhong nü qing nan* (Women over men), Shanghai: Wenhua shenghuo chubanshe, 1941, p. 133.

CONCEPTION, IMAGINATION AND
NATURAL RETRIBUTION

Belief in the power of maternal impressions was consolidated by neo-Lamarckism, as characteristics acquired during pregnancy were thought to be inheritable and hence dangerous to the foetus. Mythical stories attesting the power of woman's imagination continued to circulate in popular culture after the fall of the empire in 1911. In 1935, for instance, an article in a Beijing daily paper reported how an aged widow had given birth to a loaf of flesh suspiciously shaped 'like a bottle gourd', a monstrous conception which was no doubt the natural retribution for a dangerous solitary habit.[56] On more learned levels of culture, the female body was represented as a vulnerable entity, destined to a passive role in society by virtue of its diluted blood, smaller brain and fragile nervous system. An important shift took place after 1911, as nervous sensibility complemented the more traditional emphasis on blood in the aetiology of suffering.[57] The illness spread out from the woman's reproductive organs towards the entire body, characterised by particular qualities – vulnerability, fragility, sensibility – that were responsible for nervous disorders. The traditional notion of 'anxiety' (si) was scientised by the deployment of a new vocabulary of 'nerves' and 'neurones': according to an ABC of sexology (1928), the 'sex centre' (seqing zhongshu), thought to be part of the nervous system, could subsist in some old women, who would 'imagine sexual life'.[58]

56 'Shaoxing yi laoshuang chansheng huluxing rouqiu' (Old widow from Shaoxing gives birth to flesh loaf shaped like bottle gourd), Beiping chenbao, 5 June 1935, p. 3.
57 Neurasthenia and the scientific construction of gender differences are discussed in Dikötter, Sex, culture and modernity in China, in particular 'The passive sex: The naturalization of gender distinctions', pp. 14–61 and '"Maladie d'époque": Sexual neurasthenia', pp. 162–5.
58 Chai Fuyuan, Xingxue ABC (ABC of sexology), Shanghai: Shijie shuju, 1928, p. 46.

As in late imperial China, 'imagination' remained a dangerous activity that could precipitate vulnerable female minds into bodily decay. Wang Chengpin, addressing the issue of 'neurasthenia' (shenjing shuairuo) in aged women, thought that 'those who have sunk to this condition have recourse to unnatural practices when they are unhappy in their sex lives, or excessively indulge in imagination, trying to picture obscene postures in order to satisfy their lecherous desires.'[59] Emotions seemed to rule a precarious and unstable constitution, subjecting women to unpredictable mood changes: 'This sort of emotionalism is closely related to the changes which take place in the internal organs. Since the organisation of the internal organs – such as the ovaries, the uterus, the breasts etc. – is more complex in girls than in boys, external stimuli easily bring about vast and complex internal reactions.'[60] In a reconfiguration of humoural theories current in imperial times, in which specific organs were thought to govern different moods, modernising writers in China appropriated new scientific vocabularies to construct a close correlation between physiological changes and psychological states. The lungs were transformed under the influence of moods: they choked with grief, burst with rage and contracted with fear. Digestion was eased by bursts of joy but impeded by anger. Adrenaline ('a sort of hormone') best illustrated how women lived under the grip of nature: in extreme anger, it entered the bloodstream, raised blood pressure, increased the rate of the heartbeat and caused the organism to gather strength. Unbridled passion in particular was thought to cause havoc on the organism: 'Difficult problems and mental work should be avoided,' wrote the female authors of a popular Mirror of health for women. 'Also, novels and other

---

59 Wang Chengpin, Qingchun de xingjiaoyu (Sex education for youth), Shanghai: Xiongdi chubanshe, 1939, p. 114.
60 Zhu Yunping, Xingjiaoyu gailun (Outline of sex education), Shanghai: Shijie shuju, 1941, p. 60.

reading material which stir up passions should be forbidden, or mental decline will set in without hope of recovery'.[61]

The proposition of a close union between body and mind was consolidated by the theory of recapitulation, part of neo-Lamarckian theories of evolution. Menstruation was seen as an evolutionary throwback with dangerous consequences: 'I have seen many women who suffer from mental disorders. These disorders emerge in an extreme form during menstruation, hence even if it is a disease, normal women also have this tendency, which simply becomes more apparent in those who are diseased.'[62] Hysteria, part of an entire panoply of mental disorders that preyed upon vulnerable women, was yet another indication of the close bond between body and mind: 'Her sense of self-restraint is weak and she often harbours vain thoughts,' wrote Cao Guanlai in a popular book still displayed in some public libraries in Taiwan and Hong Kong, 'hence she easily commits crimes; she will offend the law with cruel criminal acts while she is in a state of somnolence. The changes are particularly acute when she has her periods or when she is pregnant, so one should be especially vigilant.'[63] Gynaecological treatises represented women as dangerous bundles of raw nerves, ready to explode at any time. The ovaries and the womb in particular were hypersensitive, while structural extremities like the head and the 'tail' (sic) could endure intermittent waves of pain.[64]

Some booklets on foetal education (taijiao) consequently commended a strict control of emotions and discipline of gestures. Capable of unbalanced impulses, suffering from an excessive sensitivity, pregnant women had the power both to

61 Guo Renji and Li Renlin, Nüxing yangsheng jian (Mirror of health for women), Shanghai: Shangwu yinshuguan, 1928 (1st edn 1922), pp. 33–4.

62 Cao Guanlai, Qingchun shengli tan (Chats about the physiology of youth), Taibei: Zhengzhong shuju, 1982 (1st edn 1936).

63 Cao, Qingchun, p. 60.

64 Cheng Hao, Fukexue (Gynaecology), Shanghai: Shangwu yinshuguan, 1950 (9th edn; 1st edn 1939), pp. 183–6.

engender and to transmit a destructive violence which menaced foetal health. Suggestive of more traditional medical exhortations, but also reflective of social anxieties generated by modernity, medical writers warned against violent cinema images which might 'hit the eye and stir the heart' (*chumu jingxin*).[65] Any excessive excitation might contribute to a malformed baby being born. According to the popular manual entitled *Advice on Childbirth* (1933), pernicious influences were directly transmitted to the foetus via the blood: 'If the woman suffers from a psychological condition, there is an immediate influence on the blood which may stimulate the foetus. If the excitation is too powerful, abnormal uterine contractions which oppress the foetus and impede its physiological development may occur.'[66] Another health manual for pregnant women, published in 1939, highlighted the destructive power of imagination: the fear of a monster in a young girl was in itself enough actually to engender one. Tragic news should be hidden, in particular rumours about monstrous births, which might leave a lasting imprint upon the embryo.[67] Yu Fengbin, president of the prestigious Chinese Medical Association from 1920 to 1922, warned that a sudden scare felt by the mother would shock her foetus into a state of permanent epilepsy,[68] while others intoned that the child would be retarded if conception took place when the parents were tired or under the influence of alcohol.[69] The power of analogy was such that if portraits of famous people and propitious images were displayed on the

65 Song Jiazhao, *Taijiao* (Foetal education), Shanghai: Zhonghua shuju, 1914, pp. 37–9.

66 Wang Yang, *Shengyu guwen* (Advice on childbirth), Shanghai: Zhongyang shuju, 1933, pp. 53–4.

67 Su Yizhen, *Funü shengyu lun* (About women bearing children), Shanghai: Zhonghua shuju, 1922, pp. 27–8.

68 Yu Fengbin, *Geren weisheng pian* (Personal hygiene), Shanghai: Shangwu yinshuguan, 1931 (1st edn 1917), p. 128.

69 Zhao Shifa, *Geren weishengxue* (Personal hygiene), Nanjing: Nanjing shudian, 1933, p. 198.

walls of the pregnant women's room, they could contribute to ensuring virtuous offspring.[70] Far from envisaging the exteriority of a body which remained separate from the soul, as in European medical discourse to the end of the nineteenth century, or on the contrary from subjectivising the individual body in a medical focus on a self which was thought to suffer from all sorts of disorders, an approach which originated in the 1880s to culminate in twentieth-century psychoanalysis, medical writers in China selectively appropriated biomedical knowledge in order to rethink somatisation in modern terms. Body and soul remained closely interwoven in a holistic approach which endowed women with the burden of responsibility over the reproductive health of the modern couple.

Traditional notions of foetal education – widespread in popular culture according to anthropological literature[71] – were repeated under the aegis of science. Reminiscent of the medicine of systematic correspondence, governed by analogical modes of construction, dependent on notions of balance and excess, the rules of foetal education appeared in feminist journals, manuals of hygiene and obstetric treatises. Advertisements proclaiming the merits of medical products in foetal education even appeared in daily newspapers. For instance, the Three Friends Nourishing Pills (*sanyou buwan*) were advertised as a modern means of enhancing foetal health in the interests of a virtuous progeny.[72] Older folk notions concerning the diet of pregnant women were reconfigured; mysterious powers of disruption were assigned to specific types of food, for instance the consumption of sparrow brain, which would result in nyctalopia (night blindness, called 'sparrow's blindness', *qiaomangyan*), or rabbit

70 Zhuang Weizhong, *Jiankangshu wenda* (Questions and answers on the art of health), Shanghai: Dahua shuju, 1934, pp. 6–11.

71 Francis L.K. Hsu, *Under the ancestors' shadow: Chinese culture and personality*, London: Routledge and Kegan Paul, 1949, p. 199.

72 See for instance the February issues of the *Xinwenbao* in 1940.

meat, which would lead naturally to a harelip.[73] Analogies of sound and form were thought to converge in the consumption of ginger, which resembled a human finger and could induce the appearance of supernumerary fingers in the baby. Ingestion of raw ginger (*shengjiang*) might cause the foetus being 'born stiff dead' (*shengjiang*).[74] Guided more by ideals of systematic correspondence than by the laws of evidence they so eagerly invoked, modernising intellectuals writing under the banner of science represented the foetal body as an intrinsic part of a holistic environment, an 'inner' potential shaped by the 'external' forces of the social milieu, from food and emotions to the climate and the seasons.

Some writers used Mendelian laws of inheritance to launch a systematic attack on the belief in the virtues of foetal education,[75] but a majority of writers welcomed it as a 'new science' that could contribute to the betterment of the 'race'.[76] On a variation of Kang Youwei's proposal for an institution in which selected women would be impregnated and medically tutored to breed superior offspring, Cai Yuanpei himself envisaged in 1922 the creation of a Foetal Education Institute (*taijiaoyuan*) in his quest for 'racial improvement': such institutes, built in traditional architecture with a touch of Greek art and located in scenic surroundings away from the polluted cities, would hide the ugly and

73 Cai Luxian, *Taichan kebing wenda* (Questions and answers about obstetric problems), Shanghai: Huadong shuju, 1937, pp. 9–11.

74 Yao Changxu, *Taichan xuzhi* (Essentials of obstetrics), Shanghai: Shangwu yinshuguan, 1929 (1st edn 1920), p. 22.

75 Chen Jianshan, *Taijiao* (Foetal education), Shanghai: Shangwu yinshuguan, 1926.

76 Wang Chuanying (tr.), 'Xin taijiao' (New foetal education), *Funü zazhi*, 4, no. 1–2 (Jan.–Feb. 1918); see also Xishen (tr.), 'Renshenzhong zhi jingshen ganying' (Spiritual impressions during pregnancy), *Funü zazhi*, 2, no. 10 (Oct. 1916), pp. 13-15; Zhu Wenying, 'Taijiao yu youshengxue' (Foetal education and eugenics), *Funü zazhi*, 17, no. 8 (Aug. 1931), pp. 11–19; see also Song Jiazhao, *Taijiao* (Foetal education), Shanghai: Zhonghua shuju, 1914; Song Mingzhi, *Taijiao* (Foetal education), Shanghai: Zhonghua shuju, 1914.

depraved products of modernity from pregnant women and allow them instead to admire paintings and sculptures of healthy nude bodies in a serene environment bathed in soothing music.[77] Another great pioneer in eugenic studies was the notorious 'sex revolutionary' Zhang Jingsheng, who proposed a 'New Foetal Education' in his book entitled *Plan for a Beautiful Society* in order to avoid the birth of infants 'shaped like monkeys, with a flat forehead, protruding jaws, flat noses and twisted ears'.[78]

Ideas of foetal education were compatible with a number of core values of modernity, in particular in their representation of embryonic growth as a controllable process, a departure from fatalistic expectations which prevailed on more popular levels of culture. While such ideas enhanced the social status of women, who were given a responsibility over the uterine environment, they also confirmed traditional gender distinctions by identifying women as the principal depositories of reproductive health. On the other hand, the ideal of gender complementarity and conjugal harmony was promoted, since it was thought to have eugenic virtues. The embryo, the mother, the conjugal couple and the nation were related in a biological bond and a common social responsibility by foetal education. The uterine space emerged in medical discourse as a domain of public interest in which the state was said to have a right to interfere. Not without resonance to the Confucian emphasis on education and self-cultivation, foetal education – finally – was part of an overall emphasis on the need to educate, instruct, reform and enlighten the nation of the necessity strictly to observe rules

77 Cai Yuanpei, 'Meiyu shishi de fangfa' (Methods to implement beautiful births) in Cai Yuanpei, *Cai Yuanpei quanji* (The complete works of Cai Yuanpei), Beijing: Zhonghua shuju, 1984, vol. 4, pp. 211–16.

78 Zhang Jingsheng, *Mei de shehui zuzhifa* (Plan for a beautiful society), Beijing: Beixin shuju, 1926, p. 56; on other aspects of Zhang's work, see Dikötter, *Sex, culture and modernity*, pp. 42, 57–9, 76–8, 93, 141, 152 and 170.

of sexual hygiene and closely monitor reproduction in the name of a eugenic future.

THE IMPROVEMENT OF THE RACE: THE SPREAD OF EUGENIC DISCOURSE

Reproductive information for married couples, medical advice for pregnant women, even sex knowledge for young people figured prominently in the discursive explosion which marked early republican China. After the Guomindang came to power in 1927, the theoretical concern with national revival became one of the main political and social priorities of the central government. Public health campaigns and sanitation movements, from the implementation of smallpox vaccination to the construction of urban sewer systems, were linked to the idea of regenerating the nation, since it was thought that improvements in the environment could be passed on to future generations and gradually lead to racial improvement. In this modern vision of national revival, mass education programmes in health were also undertaken, and a focus on the individual begot a new concern for health education and medical examinations of infants and children.[79] It was even planned that 'sex hygiene' and 'social medicine' should be taught in senior middle schools, although lack of adequate funds and teaching material impeded the full implementation of this aspect of mass education. The Ministry of Health planned to introduce a nation-wide service to provide health care for pregnant women in 1928. A year later, the First Midwifery School was opened in Beijing, while other maternal and child welfare initiatives appeared in other cities, notably Nanjing and Shanghai. A Child Health Institute was established in 1930

79 The following is based on Yip Ka-che, *Health and national reconstruction in nationalist China: The development of modern health services, 1928–1937*, Ann Arbor, MI: Association for Asian Studies, 1995, pp. 119–24 and 127.

and entrusted with, among other things, the task of training mothers in reproductive hygiene and carrying out prenatal examinations. In 1932 the municipal health administration of Nanjing initiated an ambitious programme to seek out expectant women and monitor their pregnancies.

If the social subject could be taught to discipline his or her reproduction, the menaces of heredity should be averted by the intervention of the state. Despite their proclaimed belief in the virtues of education, with the purpose of enlightening the population about the dangerous consequences of uncontrolled reproduction, important sectors of the educated élite, from medical experts to university teachers, believed that some categories of people were beyond the reach of reason, and that the state had a duty to curb the reproduction of those elements who could not be trusted to be sufficiently self-restrained. Proponents of eugenics claimed that breeding principles such as assortative mating and artificial selection could prevent further degeneration. 'Positive eugenics' – a term first coined by Francis Galton (1822–1911), whose portrait quickly became an emblem of modernity in many textbooks on human biology – would ensure that individuals with above-average abilities bred at a higher rate than ordinary people. 'Negative eugenics' would restrict the reproduction of inferior people; those with subnormal abilities would have to be physically prevented from perpetuating their infirmities. Mainline eugenists assumed that intellectual capacity and behavioural traits were inherited and could not be significantly enhanced by education. Those defined as being of the lowest intelligence became the main target of eugenic discourse, which campaigned for their segregation or sterilisation.

Initially referred to as 'improvement of the race' (*renzhong gailiang*), 'science of racial betterment' (*shuzhongxue*) or even 'science of intelligent descendants' (*zhesixue*), the term 'eugenics' (*youshengxue*), meaning literally 'science of superior birth', became common in republican China in the 1920s and '30s. Used in a political climate pervaded by evolutionary notions of survival and competition, the term was reminiscent of 'struggle for survival' (*youshengliebai*, meaning 'the superior win, the inferior lose'): it was homophonous with 'science of how the superior win'. Although eugenics never achieved a significant degree of institutional organisation in republican China, notions of race improvement were widespread and pervasive among professional groups, as has already been discussed in some detail elsewhere.[80] There is little evidence to show that the widespread interest in eugenic ideas was translated into actual practice before the advent of a socialist regime, although some isolated cases, such as the execution of lepers by the police in Guangdong province in the 1930s, point to a more radical approach in questions of public health during the Nanjing decade.[81]

Hereditary principles, endowing sex with a biological responsibility for future generations, were thought to highlight the need for medical intervention. Controversies over population control and race improvement in republican China were closely related to discussions of public hygiene, venereal disease and prostitution. The physical vigour and moral purity of the nation demanded the elimination of deviant practices. They were described as 'social problems' (*shehui wenti*), and the debates on sexual hygiene and venereal disease were indicative of cultural anxieties among the new professional élites of the urban centres. Thought of as a product of 'modern civilisation', syphilis in particular conjured up images of urban decay and racial decline: sex could transmit diseases, infect the body of society and threaten future genera-

80 The following section is treated in much greater detail in Frank Dikötter, 'Eugenics in Republican China', *Republican China*, 15, no. 1 (Nov. 1989), pp. 1–18, Dikötter, *Discourse of race*, chapter 6, and Dikötter, *Sex, culture and modernity*, chapter 4.
81 Carol Benedict, 'Chinese police campaigns against persons with leprosy, 1934–37', paper presented at the Annual Meeting of the Association of Asian Studies, Chicago, 14–16 March 1996.

tions.[82] Dispensaries for treating venereal disease, licensed houses to regulate prostitution, medical dossiers for the registration of infected individuals – in short, an entire disciplinary system was demanded in publications about human reproduction. By linking human reproduction to national strength, modernising élites pushed for an increased intervention of the medical professions and the state in the sexual lives of citizens. The transformation of sex into a medical category denoting degeneracy, disease and contamination was also part of a broader shift in emphasis towards biology and the body as the foundation for prescriptions about social order.

Representations of the family as genetic capital which needed to be properly managed were reinforced by the monster, who was thought to reveal a hidden biological defect running through the lineage. Detailed studies on family lines and lineage registers were meant to show that marriages of close blood relatives could cause severe retardation or congenital malformations in offspring, while medical discourse increasingly explained that an entire series of 'defects' could have a hereditary basis. Medical science not only made possible a much higher degree of specification of the 'abnormal', but allowed a virtually inexhaustible enumeration of 'dysgenic' births. The most arbitrary lists of 'defective elements' were compiled by some eugenists, whose uneven grasp of human biology was only matched by their willingness to curb coercively the reproduction of people defined as 'inferior'. From alcoholics and criminals to the feeble-minded and physically weak, different categories of people loosely grouped according to the vaguest of medical criteria were proposed for sterilisation, castration or exile.[83] A university

82 A more detailed discussion of STDs in China, including HIV/AIDS, appears in Frank Dikötter, 'A cultural history of sexually transmitted diseases in China' in Scott Bamber, Milton Lewis and Michael Waugh (eds), *Sex, disease, and society: A comparative history of sexually transmitted diseases and HIV/AIDS in Asia and the Pacific*, Westport, CT: Greenwood Press, 1997, pp. 67–84.
83 Examples are provided in Dikötter, *Discourse of race*, chapter 6.

textbook used after the Second World War, for instance, proposed to prevent 'idiots' (*chiyu*), 'demented people' (*kuangdian*), epileptics, those afflicted with 'loathsome' diseases, the malformed and those suffering from hereditary diseases from marrying, while people presenting minor infirmities like deafness, dumbness, blindness or baldness (*sic*) should be persuaded to undergo voluntary sterilisation.[84] A commitment to Mendelian laws was not necessary within a neo-Lamarckian approach to inheritance: even those who expressed doubts about the power of 'genes' sometimes subscribed to the idea of a marriage ban for people with contagious diseases, the mentally disturbed, the feeble-minded and even the maimed: if acquired features could be inherited, why only prevent elements with chromosomal abnormalities from degenerating the race?[85]

Such explanations supported the class bias which pervaded eugenic theories, as many modernising writers defined intellectuals as a superior 'class' (*jieji*) opposed to the inferior elements 'without intelligence' who propagated at the bottom of society. Deploring the differential birth rates between intellectuals and the lower classes, a number of popular writers advocated the eugenic control of those hordes of deficient people at the bottom of society who drained the race of its vitality, threatening to submerge the nation's fittest elements. Modernising intellectuals revealed that while the best educated and most skilled people in the cities were reducing the size of their families, the most uneducated reproduced themselves in large numbers. Public attention focused on the inverse correlations existing between fertility and social status, as 'race quality' became a keyword in an age of anxiety over the genetically unfit. Hu Buchan, among others, deplored the declining birth rate of intellectuals while

84 Hao Qinming, *Yichuanxue* (Genetics), Shanghai: Zhengzhong shuju, 1948, pp. 207–9.
85 Chen Tianbiao, *Renkou wenti yanjiu* (Research on population problems), Shanghai: Liming shuju, 1930, pp. 33–3 and 143.

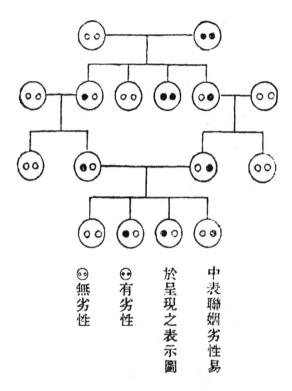

Graph illustrating transmission of 'good' and 'bad' characteristics.

expressing his apprehension about poor people: 'The streets are full of beggars, carrying each other on their backs, tramping around hand in hand; for it is true that the poorer people are, the higher their rate of reproduction.'[86] Hu even explicitly compared intellectuals in China with pure-blooded Romans in the ancient world, seeing the lower classes as no more than brutish slaves.

Social prejudice not only structured eugenic discourse, but also affected the introduction of birth control, which was heralded by some authors as a modern tool for the 'regenera-

86 Hu Buchan, *Youshengxue yu renlei yichuanxue* (Eugenics and human genetics), Taibei: Zhengzhong shuju, 1959 (1st edn 1936), p. 204.

tion of the race'[87] while others portrayed it as a contribution to 'race suicide'. For instance, Pan Guangdan predicted that inferior creatures would swamp the professional classes who practised birth control.[88] Gao Xisheng, the author of an *ABC of birth control* (1929), emphasised that 90 per cent of the children born of factory girls were 'mentally retarded' (*dineng*),[89] a dysgenic tendency which was thought to increase with the dissemination of contraceptive knowledge to the educated public. Despite these contradictory approaches to birth control, however, most writers identified the lower classes as a major problem in the eugenic regeneration of the nation.

If belief in soft inheritance was more widespread among the nationalist intellectuals eager to write in the name of science without much sustained training, even more professionally-oriented scientists who supported a strictly Mendelian approach to questions of heredity proclaimed their faith in the power of medical science to improve the race. As genetic knowledge became more common in the 1930s, the work of Weissmann, Galton and Pearson was deployed to show that genes were the carriers of physical and spiritual characteristics which could hardly be improved by changes to the environment. Even retardation and criminality were thought to run in families, as Shi Lu, author of an introduction to genetics, explained: 'Generally speaking, the family pedigree of criminals is exactly the same as the family pedigree of the feeble-minded.'[90] Other eugenists who supported a strictly Mendelian approach, including Pan Guangdan, Zhou Jianren, Chen Da and Chen Jianshan, clamoured for the proscription

87 'Ying Sanger Furen' (Welcoming Miss Sanger), *Funü zazhi*, no. 6 (June 1922), p. 3.
88 On Pan Guangdan, see Dikötter, *The discourse of race*, pp. 174–85.
89 Gao Xisheng, *Chan'er zhixian ABC* (ABC of birth control), Shanghai: Shijie shuju, 1929.
90 Shi Lu, *Yichuanxue dayi* (Outline of heredity), Shanghai: Shenzhou guoguangshe, 1931, p. 72.

of dysgenic marriages and the strict control of the reproductive capacity of those defined as unfit.[91]

However, not everybody in China believed in the regenerating virtues of eugenics, and a number of sceptical voices were raised within the field of population studies. Sun Benwen, Xu Shilian, Chen Tianbiao, Ru Song and a few others refuted the crude biological determinism of eugenic theories, criticised the capacity of IQ tests to indicate inborn intelligence, doubted whether qualities such as 'superiority' and 'inferiority' existed at birth, and generally judged the improvement of the environment to be a far more decisive factor in the amelioration of public health.[92] In 1937 Qi Sihe even criticised the use of racial categories in China, and pointed out how, in the face of ample evidence to the contrary, 'race' was a declining notion in the West.[93] Yu Jingrang, although voicing concern about the declining birth-rate of the higher classes in a booklet entitled *The improvement of the race* in 1936,[94] also publicly denounced Nazi eugenics, sterilisation policies and marriage restrictions on the so-called lower classes in a revised edition of his work ten years later.[95] However, as in other countries, many intellectuals were in favour of eugenics and few members of the educated public had the desire or opportunity to dispute what passed as expert opinion. As eugenics was popularised in the 1930s, it gave scientific credibility and respectability to attitudes, anxieties and values which were prevalent primarily if not exclusively among the formally educated levels of society.

91 The works of these authors are analysed in greater detail in Dikötter, *Discourse of race*, chapter 6.

92 Dikötter, *Discourse of race*, pp. 180–1.

93 Qi Sihe, 'Zhongzu yu minzu' (Race and nationality), *Yugong*, 7, nos 1–2–3 (April 1937), pp. 25–34.

94 Yu Jingrang, *Renzhong gailiang* (Improvement of the race), Shanghai: Zhengzhong shuju, 1947 (1st edn 1936), p. 44.

95 Ibid., preface.

Despite the reservations expressed by a number of formally trained experts in the social sciences, many nationalist intellectuals could hardly contain their rage at the thought that 'Society is still crammed with all the evil, the ugly, the false, the wicked, the scrambling, the base, the stupid, the brutish and the vexing elements of the human race, filled with all the bad phenomena that could lead a superior person to commit suicide.'[96] From proposals for eugenic laboratories at the provincial level and special villages, where people with perfect brains and ideal bodies could be bred in order to generate the future 'model race', to plans for the 'forcible elimination' of entire categories of people judged deficient, such as sex criminals, the incurably sick, the feebleminded, and those afflicted with hereditary diseases, some writers did not shrink from upholding the Nazi experiments as a medically viable path to a eugenic future.[97] If the more fanatical voices did not reach beyond the pages of specialised journals, others were taken seriously in government circles. Zhang Junjun, a prolific author on the question of race improvement, gained the support of top officials for his 'Draft for the Implementation of Shaanxi's Race Reform'.[98] It included a plan for an Institute of Race Reform, in which the eugenics department would be responsible for approving marriages, encouraging 'superior births' and preventing 'unhealthy' unions in which one of the partners was feebleminded, mentally disordered, afflicted with a communicable disease, physically weak, tubercular or 'criminally inclined'. Shao Lizi, governor of Shaanxi province in 1933–6, endorsed Zhang's document. Other enthusiastic supporters included Zhang Xueliang, once the most powerful warlord in the north of

96 Xia Yuzhong, 'Shuzhongxue yu jiaoyu' (Eugenics and education), *Xinjiaoyu*, 2, no. 4 (Dec. 1919), p. 395.
97 Wei Juxian, 'Zhongguo minzu qiantu zhi shi de kaocha' (Study on the future of the Chinese race), *Qiantu*, 1, no. 10 (Oct. 1933), pp. 17–18.
98 Zhang Junjun, *Zhongguo minzu zhi gaizao* (The reform of the Chinese race), Shanghai: Zhonghua shuju, 1937 (1st edn 1935).

China, then deputy commander-in-chief of operations against the communists in the north-west; Pan Gongzhan, an influential journalist and publisher, member of the Central Executive Committee of the Guomindang and future vice-minister of information; Cai Yuanpei, founder and president of the prestigious Academia Sinica; Chen Lifu, head of the organisation department of the Guomindang, and other high-ranking officials. Eugenic ideas were of course fostered by the Guomindang, whose own New Life Movement was partly inspired by a preoccupation with a 'strong race and a strong nation'.[99]

The Japanese invasion plunged the country into a pro-longed war that pushed plans for race reform into the back-ground. The Second World War, followed by the civil war between the Communist Party and the Guomindang from 1945 to 1949, was the main reason why eugenic ideas did not achieve institutional form. The Committee for the Study of Population Policies, organised by the Ministry of Social Affairs in 1941, was the first official attempt to approach eugenics systematically. It recommended the segregation of physically and mentally handicapped persons from the nor-mal population for what was called 'cultural advancement and racial rejuvenation'. Because people were recognised as being unequally endowed, the report advocated a differential birth-rate: 'Thus viewed', said the report, 'some individuals may have children, others not.' The committee – whose members included Chen Changheng, Chen Da and Pan Guangdan – also encouraged the use of sterilisation for the racial rejuvenation of the country and recommended that '(s)teps should be taken to segregate persons of heredi-tary defects, physical or mental, from the normal popu-lation.'[100]

99 Jiang Zhongzheng (Jiang Jieshi), *Xinshenghuo yundong* (The New Life Movement), Shanghai: Zhengzhong shuju, 1935, pp. 27, 41.
100 Chen Ta, *Population in modern China*, New York: Octagon Books, 1974, pp. 76–7.

Similar developments took place in other countries, as has been documented in the enormous secondary literature produced in recent years. Eugenics was a fundamental aspect of some of the most important cultural and social movements of the interwar period, intimately linked to ideologies of 'race', nation and sex, inextricably meshed with population control, social hygiene, state hospitals and the welfare state. As a growing body of research shows, in Germany the Nazi regime translated its racial ideology into official policy by systematically persecuting Jews, Gypsies, mentally and physically handicapped people, and homosexuals.[101] However, until recently the historiographical focus on the most extreme expressions of race improvement tended to perpetuate a one-sided representation which ignored the multifarious dimensions and extraordinary appeal of eugenics to different social and political groups. Far from being a politically conservative and scientifically spurious set of beliefs which remained confined to the Nazi era, eugenics belonged to the political vocabulary of almost every significant modernising force between the two World Wars.[102] For example, eugenic programs and sterilisation laws were part of an emerging welfare

101 Peter Weingart, Jörgen Kroll and Kurt Bayertz, *Rasse, Blut und Gene. Geschichte der Eugenik und Rassenhygiene in Deutschland*, Frankfurt-am-Main: Suhrkamp, 1988 (points at continuities with debates on genetic therapy today, pp. 670–84); Michael Burleigh and Wolfgang Wippermann, *The racial state: Germany 1933–1945*, Cambridge University Press, 1991; Robert N. Proctor, *Racial hygiene: Medicine under the Nazis*, Cambridge, MA: Harvard University Press, 1988; and Paul J. Weindling, *Health, race and German politics between national unification and Nazism, 1870–1945*, Cambridge University Press, 1989. On eugenics and euthanasia, see Hans-Walter Schmuhl, *Rassenhygiene, Nationalsozialismus, Euthanasie*, Göttingen: Vandenhoeck und Ruprecht, 1987.
102 Three recent articles provide useful overviews of the field, namely Robert Nye, 'The rise and fall of the eugenics empire: Recent perspectives on the impact of bio-medical thought in modern society', *Historical Journal*, 36, no. 3 (1993), pp. 687–700; P.J. Pauly, 'Review article: The eugenics industry – Growth or restructuring?', *Journal of the History of Biology*, 26, no. 1 (spring 1993), pp. 131–45; Frank Dikötter, 'Race culture: Recent perspectives on the history of eugenics', *American Historical Review*, 103, no. 2 (April 1998), pp. 467–78.

system in Denmark, Finland, Norway and Sweden.[103] Individuals alleged to suffer from mental retardation or mental illness became the main targets of eugenic practices in these countries from the 1930s onwards. Despite a legal insistence on voluntary sterilisation, the lack of ability to make a legally valid approval by individuals judged to be mentally disturbed generally led to the operation being performed without consent. Denmark was the first Scandinavian country to pass a sterilisation law in 1929, the result of official efforts to implement eugenic policies which had started after the accession to power of the first Labour government in 1924. Support for reform eugenics continued up to the 1950s: initially pushed by the minister of justice and later of social affairs, eugenic sterilisation was presented as a fundamental aspect of an enviable social welfare state. Other countries in Scandinavia passed similar laws, pushed by government officials and medical doctors in charge of psychiatric hospitals and institutions for the mentally retarded.

In the United States, as is well documented, a number of states actually passed sterilisation laws and limited marriage selection.[104] Less well known is the fact that eugenics also thrived in relatively isolated and provincial parts of that country, as a small number of determined individuals influenced eugenic legislation in the Deep South.[105] Practising physicians blamed the 'insane' and the 'feeble-minded' for a variety of social problems. Invoking the language of science, to which they themselves contributed preciously little, medical authorities proposed marriage restrictions, sexual segregation and compulsory sterilisation to curb the reproduction of people with presumed dysgenic traits. Introduced during the

103 Gunnar Broberg and Nils Roll-Hansen (eds), *Eugenics and the welfare state: Sterilization policy in Denmark, Sweden, Norway, and Finland*, East Lansing: Michigan State University Press, 1996.

104 D.J. Kevles, *In the name of eugenics: Genetics and the use of human heredity*, New York: Alfred Knopf, 1985.

105 Edward J. Larson, *Sex, race, and science: Eugenics in the Deep South*, Baltimore: Johns Hopkins University Press, 1996.

first two decades of this century, eugenic statutes providing for the sexual segregation of individuals defined as 'unfit' in state institutions were passed in all states of the region between 1918 and 1920. Moves in favour of sterilisation continued unabated in several states up until the Second World War, followed by a movement of repudiation and withdrawal from eugenic practices.

Although eugenic laws were also passed in other countries (including Switzerland), they were resisted in France, Britain and the Netherlands. In Britain, leading scientists like J.B.S. Haldane, Julian Huxley, Lancelot Hogben and Herbert Jennings turned against eugenics and denounced the race and class prejudice it cultivated.[106] If the decline in eugenics within scientific circles often preceded Nazism,[107] the cruelty of German policies eventually led to a strong reaction, supported by a long-standing and influential anti-eugenic coalition among people of both secular and religious backgrounds.[108] In the Netherlands, eugenics remained a marginal movement from the very start, as widespread resistance was expressed against the medical regulation of reproduction and state intervention in the family. A biologising vision that reduced human life to a hereditary mechanism was also attacked, while a long tradition of charitable aid combined with objections from the catholic church to contraception to form a strong movement of opposition to eugenics. Equally important was the traditional reticence of the government itself to intervene in the private life of its citizens, as the state in the Netherlands traditionally viewed the family as a sacrosanct entity that should not be interfered with or intruded upon.[109] Open democracies with a vibrant civil society, such

106 D.J. Kevles, *In the name of eugenics: Genetics and the use of human heredity*, New York: Alfred Knopf, 1985, p. 120.
107 Elazar Barkan, *The retreat of scientific racism: Changing concepts of race in Britain and the United States between the two World Wars*, Cambridge University Press, 1992, pp. 260–76.
108 Kevles, *In the name of eugenics*, p. 118.
109 Jan Noordman, *Om de kwaliteit van het nageslacht. Eugenetika in Nederland,*

as Britain and the Netherlands, were generally less inclined to adopt extreme eugenic proposals than contemporary authoritarian regimes in Germany, Italy and China. Historians of medicine have demonstrated the existence of a close link between eugenic theories and Mendelian genetics, in particular in countries like England and Germany. Neo-Lamarckian approaches to inheritance, however, were not incompatible with eugenic discourse, as is clearly demonstrated in the case of Russia and Brazil, two countries which also harboured strident advocates of eugenic sterilisation.[110] Proponents of neo-Lamarckism claimed that undesirable traits like alcoholism were acquired in one generation and passed on to the next: the belief in the inheritance of acquired features did not need to be based on a genealogical analysis to demonstrate that a trait followed Mendelian laws. Environmental determinism, rather than biological determinism, was used to advocate the sterilisation of particular categories of people. France has been characterised as the 'home of neo-Lamarckian eugenics', an emphasis which is explained partly because of the pronounced concern over the declining birth-rate and fears of underpopulation. While eugenists in France did not support Mendelian laws, they still called for the elimination of dysgenic elements, although they generally preferred to encourage the propagation of the 'fit' and the improvement of the health of the 'unfit'. In con-

1900–1950, Nijmegen: SUN, 1989; see also P. van Praag, Het bevolkingsvraagstuk in Nederland. Ontwikkeling van standpunten en opvattingen (1918–1940), Deventer: Van Loghum Slaterus, 1976, pp. 97–105; H. Biervliet, 'Biologisme, racisme en eugenetiek in de antropologie en sociologie van de jaren dertig' in F. Bovenkerk et al. (eds), Toen en thans. De sociale wetenschappen in de jaren dertig en nu, Baarn: Ambo, 1978, pp. 208–35.

110 Nancy L. Stepan, 'Eugenics in Brazil, 1917–1940' and Mark B. Adams, 'Eugenics in Russia, 1900–1940' in Mark B. Adams (ed.), The wellborn science: Eugenics in Germany, France, Brazil and Russia, Oxford University Press, 1990, pp. 110–216; see also Dain Borges, '"Puffy, ugly, slothful and inert": Degeneration in Brazilian social thought, 1880–1940', Journal of Latin American Studies, 25 (1993), pp. 235–56.

trast to researchers in Germany and Britain, French eugenists did not produce significant biological research or statistical studies; as in China, it was part of the vocabulary of most political groups, from far left to extreme right, as many intellectuals shared a concern over modernity, a sense of nationalism and an expectation that the government would reform society. But in France, widespread reluctance to interfere in the private lives of families, opposition from religious and liberal groups, and the sense among family doctors of their professional duty to respect the confidentiality of their patients combined to marginalise eugenic proposals.[111]

Republican China combined Mendelian genetics with neo-Lamarckian approaches to inheritance in a holistic approach which stressed the interdependence of nature with nurture and the subordination of the individual to the nation. Just as the absence of a clear boundary between body and mind characterised medical discourse, no clear distinctions were made between socially undesirable features and genetic disorders. In a climate of distrust of liberal individualism and of pluralistic democracy, and in the absence of a religion which disregarded bodily attributes in favour of a paramount spirit, the desire for control over reproduction could only gain strength with the advent of a one-party state in 1949.

111 William H. Schneider, *Quality and quantity: The quest for biological regeneration in twentieth-century France*, Cambridge University Press, 1990; Anne Carol, *Histoire de l'eugénisme en France. Les médecins et la procréation, XIXe-XXe siècle*, Paris: Seuil, 1995; Pierre-André Taguieff, 'Eugénisme ou décadence? L'exception française', *Ethnologie Française*, no. 24, no. 1 (Jan.–March 1994), pp. 81–103.

4

'INFERIOR BIRTHS': EUGENICS IN THE PEOPLE'S REPUBLIC OF CHINA

INTRODUCTION

Medical knowledge in republican China was articulated around a multiplicity of points in the social field and anchored in various cultural locations. In the absence of strong professional associations, no unified interest group governed medical discourse; instead it attracted social reformers, professional writers, sex educators, university professors and political ideologues, as well as medical experts. Even after the establishment of a central government in 1927, when the intellectual establishment with a modern education gained more power and prestige, the dispersed nature of medical knowledge did not fundamentally change. Unlike the situation in some European countries in the 1930s, where medical theories advocating the strict regulation of human reproduction were generated by an integrated scientific community under state control, few links can be established in republican China between the interests of the state and the discursive practices of a loose association of more or less independent intellectuals.[1] Even if maternal and child health was relatively high on the agenda of the Nationalist government, medical authorities had more urgent priorities than the eugenic amelioration of the population. They were confronted with many serious diseases such as cholera, smallpox, typhoid fever, tuberculosis and leprosy, which remained rampant well into the 1950s.

Public health became a major political issue in the People's Republic of China (PRC), and a number of health cam-

---

1 See Dikötter, *Sex, culture and modernity*, in particular the introduction.

paigns and sanitation movements were started immediately after the communist victory in 1949. The Ministry of Health organised teams to investigate the epidemiological state of the country and work out strategies to prevent and treat the most common diseases. In contrast to the republican period, moreover, the central government was able to curb intellectual diversity and exert effective control over the medical profession. Science, medicine and the state became closely linked as the socialist regime consolidated its power in the PRC's first decade. Moreover, in its emphasis on political allegiance rather than professional expertise, the socialist regime denounced large sectors of the medical field, and many experts came under severe attack in the wake of the anti-rightist campaign of 1957.

Efforts to discredit eugenics on Marxist terms had appeared sporadically in the 1930s,[2] but only after the communist victory in 1949 was the class bias of eugenic discourse systematically condemned. Zhou Jianren, science-editor of the Commercial Press and brother of the famous writer Lu Xun, author of numerous pamphlets advocating eugenics in the 1930s, became an official mouthpiece of the party and published a radical critique of eugenics and racial discrimination, which it portrayed as imperialist tools of domination over the working class.[3] Pan Guangdan, who had made eugenics a household word in China, was singled out for severe criticism during the anti-rightist campaign in 1957. Genetics and physical anthropology were also denounced as 'bourgeois science'. As in the Soviet Union, Lysenko's doctrine became dominant in the 1950s and '60s while Mendelian laws of inheritance and T.H. Morgan's chromosome theory were rejected for ideological reasons. Sup-

2 Ru Song, 'Ping youshengxue yu huanjinglun de lunzheng' (Reviewing the controversy between eugenics and environment), *Ershi shiji*, 1, no. 1 (Feb. 1931), pp. 57–124.
3 Zhou Jianren, *Lun youshengxue yu zhongzu qishi* (About eugenics and racial discrimination), Beijing: Sanlian shudian, 1950.

porters of Lysenko argued that acquired characteristics could be inherited while outer environmental influences could be manipulated so as to alter an organism's features. Genetic research received only limited support during the years of Lysenkoism, although some work on DNA and inherited disorders was carried out by the Dalian Hospital, the Shanghai Hospital and the Anshan Eastern Steel Hospital.[4]

In the onslaught of the Cultural Revolution, teachers, researchers and scientists were repeatedly persecuted, harassed and tortured, as Red Guard organisations inflicted sustained damage on research centres and educational institutions. Although no precise figures are available, the trial of the Gang of Four indicates that at least 500 professors and associate professors in the medical colleges and institutes under the Ministry of Health were 'falsely charged and persecuted'.[5] Up till the death of Mao Zedong in 1976, the emphasis on class background rather than on scholarly promise continued to disrupt urban medical care, as nurses were promoted to work as doctors even as doctors were demoted to empty bedpans and clean windows.[6] However, eugenic theories briefly surfaced during this period of turmoil as political publications stressed the biological heri-

---

4 Laurence A. Schneider, 'Learning from Russia: Lysenkoism and the fate of genetics in China, 1950–1986' in Merle Goldman and Denis F. Simon (eds), *Science and technology in post-Mao China*, Cambridge, MA: Harvard University Press, 1989, pp. 45–65; see also Laurence A. Schneider, *Lysenkoism in China: Proceedings of the 1956 Qingdao Genetics Symposium*, Armonk, NY: M.E. Sharpe, 1986.

5 Harry Harding, 'The Cultural Revolution: China in turmoil, 1966–1969' in Roderick MacFarquhar and John K. Fairbank (eds), *Cambridge History of China*, vol. 15: *The People's Republic*, part 2: *Revolutions within the Chinese revolution, 1966–1982*, Cambridge University Press, 1991, pp. 211–12.

6 Martin King Whyte, 'Urban life in the People's Republic' in MacFarquhar and Fairbank, *Cambridge History of China, Revolutions within the Chinese revolution*, p. 721.

tability of class attitudes.[7] Blood-lineage theories were occasionally deployed to prove that the best communists were
'born red', and traditional proverbs such as 'a phoenix begets
phoenixes, a wolf begets wolves' were in vogue for some
time.[8]

The damage inflicted on medical research and public
health was only reversed after the accession of Deng
Xiaoping to power in 1978. Medical experts and population
specialists were put into powerful positions of responsibility
as official policies aimed at the limitation of births were initiated by the government. Although the one-child family programme, by which the government only in exceptional
circumstances allows parents to have more than one or occasionally two children, is relatively well known,[9] an important
component of these policies has been the improvement of
the quality of new-born babies. The control of the 'quality'
of births has been regarded in China as being no less important than the control of 'quantity': both have regularly been
heralded as the twin goals in the control of reproduction
since 1978.

Official approaches to reproductive health since 1978
serve many practical functions which could be interpreted
favourably as a contribution to the reduction of disabilities: a
commitment to modern technology in prenatal care, a focus

7 On theories of 'natural redness', see Gordon White, *The politics of class and class
origin: The case of the Cultural Revolution*, Canberra: Australian National
University, 1976, and Richard Curt Krauss, 'Class conflict and the vocabulary of
social analysis', *China Quarterly*, 69 (March 1977), pp. 54–74.
8 See for instance Gao Yuan, *Born red: A chronicle of the Cultural Revolution*,
Stanford University Press, 1987, pp. 84, 113, 119, 122, 209.
9 Some useful works include Judith Banister, *China's changing population*, Stanford
University Press, 1987; Penny Kane, *China and the one-child family*, New York:
M. Russell, 1984; Peng Xizhe, *Demographic transition in China: Fertility trends since
the 1950s*, Oxford: Clarendon Press, 1991; Song Chien, *Population control in
China: Theory and applications*, New York: Praeger, 1985; Susan Greenhalgh,
'State society links: Political dimensions of population policies and programs,
with special reference to China', *Working Paper 18*, New York: Population
Council, 1990.

on infant and maternal health care, an effort to provide medical information on genetic disorders, an attempt to strengthen support systems for disabled people are different aspects of population policies and health programmes which in many developed countries are considered perfectly legitimate. The strain on scarce economic resources of families with disabled individuals as well as the desire to achieve better levels of child health are also issues which the government seeks to address in its current policies. Taken separately, many of these concerns have few overt eugenist implications. As in the interwar period in Europe, however, a variety of different issues, including birth control, sex education, infant health care and prenatal screening techniques, are articulated within a eugenic frame which is prominent in its denial of personal choice. Even apparently non-eugenist interests, such as improved care for the handicapped, are often embedded within an approach which puts the health of the collectivity above the needs of individuals. Eugenics provides an overarching rationale for a range of reproductive and demographic concerns which are constrained by a policy which prioritises the needs of broad collectivities of interests such as 'the state', 'the economy' or 'future generations' over the possible desires and choices of individuals.

During the first conference of the China Genetics Institute in 1978, it was proposed that eugenic research be made a priority, and this was widely supported by medical experts and government officials. Besides government directives and provincial laws, a number of research centres, monitoring units and specialised hospitals dedicated to the improvement of the population's quality have also appeared in the post-Mao era. This development has been closely linked to the government's focus on eugenics, which culminated in a nation-wide eugenics law in 1995, and medical experts and official circles have adopted a number of new measures to improve child and maternal health care. Educational programmes aimed at young couples and pregnant women have also attempted to increase the medical understanding of reproductive health. On the basis of more than a hundred publications on human reproduction, encompassing both popular advice manuals and learned medical treatises, the first part of this chapter analyses the medical discourse on reproductive health in general and birth defects in particular. The second part focuses on the meanings of eugenic legislation and reproductive health in China since 1978. The social and ethical implications of an eugenic approach are briefly addressed in the conclusion to this chapter.

AIR, WATER AND FOOD: THE FOETUS AND THE ENVIRONMENT

The economic reforms and population policies implemented since 1978 have created the conditions for a greater acceptance of eugenic discourse. New publishing houses in pursuit of a profitable share in an expanding market release countless health manuals for popular consumption. Primers on sex education, pamphlets on reproductive health and handbooks of marital advice have flooded the market,[10] both reflecting and shaping the concerns of consumers eager for better knowledge in reproductive matters. A prolific medical discourse has responded to the public's concern for a child who is both healthy and virtuous or even for a genetically improved line of descent. As eugenic discourse is conflated with concerns oriented towards infant and maternal health care, it finds a large consensus among the more formally educated sectors of the population. Health manuals also thrive on popular anxieties about the health and develop-

---

10 For a general introduction to this type of literature, see Harriet Evans, 'Defining difference: The "scientific" construction of gender and sexuality in the People's Republic of China', *Signs*, 20, no. 2 (Winter 1995), pp. 357–94 and Harriet Evans, *Women and sexuality in China*, Cambridge: Polity Press, 1997.

ment of the single child, as many parents have become a ready audience for eugenic theories.

In a context of limited knowledge about basic reproductive health, popular medical publications enable ordinary people, especially women, to achieve minimal standards of hygiene. Advice on the female cycle, menstruation, sexual intercourse, pregnancy and delivery are provided with the aim of increasing reproductive health and improving offspring. Because access to sex education was minimal till the late 1970s, these publications also fulfil a practical function by allowing prospective parents to gain a better understanding of conception, pregnancy and giving birth, including human sexuality, reproductive disorders and inherited diseases. Given the very low levels of public awareness, the commitment from medical specialists and popular writers to providing readers with basic information contrasts strongly with earlier decades, when similar matters were only discussed in a peripheral way.[11] Medical publications encourage parents to take measures which could contribute to the production of healthier offspring. Many of these objectives no doubt correspond to the daily needs of ordinary people, who are as keen as parents in developed countries to produce healthy babies. However, at the same time eugenic advice on reproductive health is considerably constrained by prejudice and ignorance. The medical knowledge provided is structured by cultural, social and political values which portray the individual as an organic part of a broader collectivity: rather than enabling parents to make informed choices, medical knowledge stresses the duties and responsibilities of individuals in the achievement of a eugenic future. Human reproduction is seen as a biological mechanism which can be eugenically enhanced thanks to proper medical knowledge. This vision is further strengthened by attributing causal power to pathogenic agents: an ontological conception of disease stresses how pathological agents, whether germs,

11 Evans, *Women and sexuality in China*.

microbes or toxins, can attack a weak pregnant woman.
A holistic approach also consolidates the link between biological retribution and social disorder, as birth defects are
seen to occur when the pregnant woman has failed to protect herself against the teratogenic power of spiritual and
physical forces. Not only are women thought to be particularly vulnerable to outside forces, but they are also singled
out as a site for the control of reproductive health.

In a holistic approach to the human body, both environment and heredity are represented as potential sources of
danger to the foetus. Specialised medical treatises and popular health manuals stress that hereditary disorders are trig-
gered into activity by the environment, and enjoin the
couples to monitor their surroundings strictly in the interests
of foetal health. The environment hides poisons, chemicals
and radiations which can attack the human body. Military
metaphors are part of a strong ontological conception of pollution, in which invisible chemical particles are said to be
capable of 'assaulting' or 'invading' the human body to cause
genetic mutations and permanently alter the human gene
pool. A vision of assault is very much part of a retributive
tradition in which malevolent forces of nature have been
unleashed by human interference. Causal power is attributed
to the environment, which has been degraded by modernity
and strikes back at the very roots of human life: polluted air,
water and food can all induce malformations in the foetus.
As in late imperial China, the quality of the air is identified
as a central element in the aetiology of health. Disorders in
the air, climate and seasons are thought to be important
causes of illness. 'Air' is now seen as a quantifiable substance
that can be expressed in a chemical formula. As air pollution
is seen as a retribution for modernity, the causality of illness
is expressed in terms of a specific agent: 'chemicals' or
'toxins' act as 'germs' and 'microbes' in their strategy of
'assault' on the human body.

Health pamphlets emphasise that sprawling cities corrupt
the air, engender toxins and spawn pollution. The health of

the individual is linked to a particular way of life: a causal chain is established between illness and morality, as biological disorders are explained as a consequence of a breakdown in social order and human conduct. Health manuals express a sense of alienation, since modernity has irremediably corrupted the very basis of life: air and water are no longer 'natural', just as mankind itself has lost its 'purity'. Modernity has engendered its own reflection in the monster, as artificial radiation and chemical elements can penetrate the womb and cause mutations and malformations. While the real dangers of chemical contamination and industrial pollution should not be underestimated, the medical fears which appear in these health manuals are very much guided by social anxieties. The border between 'natural' and 'chemical' products is in itself a cultural construct, since 'chemicals' also appear in unaltered products, such as toxins in the mould *aspergillus flavus* which forms on peanuts and is more dangerous than many toxins produced by the chemical industry. Compounds known to contribute to cancer are also found in popular ingredients of herbal remedies, for instance comfrey and sassafras. Social anxieties often focus on the dangers engendered by modernity, and even television is represented as a potential threat to maternal and foetal health, since it emits X-rays which can induce mutations in the structure of DNA. The large quantity of positive ions emitted by the television set are said to cause headaches and nausea, possibly leading to miscarriage or birth defects.[12]

In the holistic universe constructed by medical knowledge, the boundaries between the foetus and the environment are porous and fragile. The foetus is inexorably part of a larger environment in so far as the individual belongs to a collectivity. It 'listens' to external sounds: the rumbling from the mother's stomach, the rushing of blood through the arteries, the endless pounding of the heart – all these noises

12 Weng Xiayun, *Jihua shengyu yu yousheng 200 wen* (200 questions about birth control and eugenics), Beijing: Jindun chubanshe, 1992, p. 93.

are claimed to structure the environment of the foetus. The deployment of ultrasonic detectors is not only a symbolic transgression of a permeable boundary between foetus and environment: constructing the conditions of their own objectivity, new medical technologies demonstrate that the foetus 'reacts' (*fanying*) to 'external stimuli' (*waijie ciji*) which invade its uterine space, frequently moving when a car honks, curling up when a door is slammed or kicking its feet when the mother has a quarrel. Rather than presenting mere factual observations, health manuals use medical knowledge to instil a sense of reproductive responsibility in pregnant mothers.

In their discussion of the relationship between food and health, medical experts rearticulate traditional notions of 'balance' and 'excess' in modernising terms. Notions of 'heat' (*re*) and 'cold' (*leng*) reappear in a new configuration based on a biomedical vocabulary of 'energy', 'calories' and 'vitamins'. 'Hot' food should be avoided in favour of bland (*dan*) flavours. The need for balance and harmony is most clearly represented in dire warnings against the dangers of *pianshi*. A selfish desire which overlooks the needs of the foetus in favour of individual pleasure, a disturbing indulgence dictated by whim rather than by reason, a personal weakness that should be eliminated in favour of a disciplined approach to diet, *pianshi* is characterised by an excessive partiality for one type of food. The pregnant woman's diet should be balanced in 'nutrients' (*yingyangsu*) and 'vitamins' (*weishengsu*), those invisible components that determine whether food is 'harmful' or 'useful' to the human body. Foods altered and corrupted by modernity are denounced as potential threats to the foetus. For instance, canned food is proscribed, since it is 'artificially engineered' in taste, flavour and colour. Health manuals focus on concrete chemical elements like additives or preservatives to represent processed food products as the symbol of modernity's dangerous manipulation of nature. In a reminder of traditional warnings about 'heat' and 'cold', it is claimed that ice-cream and cold soft-drinks – interpreted

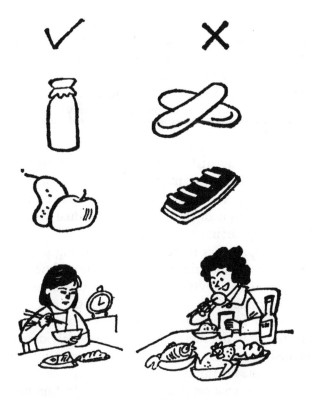

Good and bad dietary habits during pregnancy.

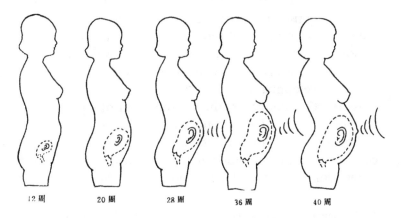

The foetus's increased awareness of the outer world.

by some writers as signs of a dangerous drift away from self-restraint towards self-indulgence – lower the resistance of the immune system.[13] The chemical elements – messengers of death – accumulate inside the body, affect the development of the foetus and lead to birth defects. An entire range of 'artificial' foods symbolise modern society's unwholesome life-style. Manipulated and altered products represent an artificial way of life imposed on alienated individuals by the rampant shopping malls and anonymous department stores brought into being by modernity. Medical discourse thus continuously makes simultaneous statements connecting the spiritual alienation of the modern individual with the bio-logical estrangement of his offspring.

Similar approaches to bodily health during pregnancy are popular in many societies and shared by very different groups of people: they invariably, but not universally, portray women as vulnerable creatures who bear the main burden of responsibility for reproductive health. Comparable ideas can also be found in the literature of advice widely distributed in developed countries, as even a cursory perusal of texts pub-lished by the Natural Childbirth Trust or the Active Childbirth Association in Britain reveals. In Europe and the United States, medical knowledge is theoretically intended to facilitate the reproductive choices of parents, but in prac-tice may be used to assign reproductive duties to women in the name of science. All too often, a woman ceases to be a person as soon as she becomes pregnant: considered a carrier of a baby, she is made to feel responsible for every aspect of a foetus's development.

As in other countries, the consumption of cigarettes and alcohol, before and after conception, is said to lead to foetal malformations or mental retardation. A woman who con-ceives in a state of alcoholic intoxication will beget a mental-ly retarded child: the alcohol absorbed in the blood is first

13 Wu Shuming, 'Xiandai shenghuo yu yousheng' (Contemporary life and eugenics), *Renkou yu yousheng*, 1993, no. 6, p. 10.

transformed into acetic aldehyde and then into acetic acid by
the liver, a process involving the production of metabolic
particles (*daixie wuzhi*) which not only are capable of causing
considerable harm to the liver, the brain and the heart, but
also affect germ cells: 'Conception after drinking can cause
delay in the development of the foetus, which may become a
retardant [*zhili dixia*], a cretin [*daiben*] or even an idiot
[*baichi*]. Consequently, for the sake of the normal development of future generations, one should not indulge in long
bouts of drinking or conceive after having consumed alcohol.'[14] The father too should restrain his consumption of
alcohol and cigarettes, since both can alter the germ cells in
his sperm, directly jeopardising the genetic fitness of his offspring.

Health manuals also support restrictions on marital age,
and produce statistics demonstrating that the incidence of
birth defects increases in pregnant women above thirty years
of age, but that girls under twenty are also 5% more at risk of
giving birth to a baby with a disorder than women in the
twenty-four to twenty-nine age-group. Similar ideas, as
noted above, are current in many developed countries. They
can be used to portray young mothers as morally and medically deviant, or even to restrict access to social support for
teenage mothers in welfare states. Few developed countries,
however, have passed the stringent marriage laws and population policies which allow the state in the PRC to implement these ideas.

The legal restrictions on marriage between young people
are thought to be founded on natural laws, since the bodies
of 'adolescents' – a medical category encompassing all individuals from puberty to marriage and represented as an
unstable and dangerous stage in the biological life-cycle[15] –
are thought to be not yet fully developed: for instance, in

14 Fang Fang, *Yousheng yu youyu* (Eugenics and quality childbirth), Beijing:
Renmin chubanshe, 1991, p. 51.
15 On the medical construction of 'adolescence', see Evans, *Women*, pp. 56–81.

young girls the pelvis has not entirely calcified, and because the foetus will absorb great quantities of calcium from the young mother, she may suffer from malformations in the bones or overexertion of the muscles, influencing in turn the development of the foetus. Adolescent mothers can also suffer from high blood-pressure, rheumatic fever, heart disease and renal problems. To establish an analogy between the shape of the sperm and the physical appearance of the foetus, it is claimed that adolescent men suffer from a low sperm count, a low quality of semen, disfigured sperm or chromosomal abnormalities, leading to a high risk of fathering malformed, retarded or otherwise handicapped children.[16] Entitled 'Semen, a eugenic capital', one article repeats in modernising terms the traditional restrictions necessary to nurture what is called 'superior sperm'.[17]

While government restrictions on early marriage are based on medical arguments which enjoy great currency in many countries, other ideas seem to be more directly indebted to indigenous notions of reproductive health. In the same way as traditional almanacs indicated the favourable and unfavourable days for human conception, a new literature of advice supports a holistic notion of a resonance between microcosm and macrocosm. The traditional emphasis on the influence of the seasons on the human body is reconfigured into the scientific notion of a biological clock (shengwuzhong), thought to synchronise the body with the environment.[18] Three separate biological clocks with different cycles are claimed to be responsible for intelligence (a cycle

16 Su Ping and Hou Dongmin, Youshengxue gailun (Introduction to eugenics), Beijing: Renmin daxue chubanshe, 1994, p. 299.

17 Zhang Yanlong, 'Jingzi, yousheng zhi ben' (Semen, a eugenic capital), Renkou yu yousheng, 1994, no. 6, p. 5.

18 For instance Song Weimin and Lu Yuelian, Renti shengwuzhong qutan (Interesting stories about the human body's biological clock), Shanghai: Zhongyi xueyuan chubanshe, 1990; Song Weimin and Lu Yuelian, Shengwuzhong yangsheng (The biological clock and the nourishment of life), Tianjin: Tianjin kexue jishu chubanshe, 1990.

of thirty-three days), physical strength (twenty-three days) and mood (twenty-eight days). In order to engender a superior child, the couple are urged to take care to conceive at the very moment when the biological clock has reached its peak. The moment of conception should ideally coincide with the peak of the biological clock in both parents, calculated on the basis of their birthdays: on 20 February 1982, a girl born on 24 August 1955 would enter her 9650th day, corresponding to the fourteenth day of the intelligence cycle, the eighteenth of the mood cycle and the thirteenth of the strength cycle. Conception on that day with an equally attuned partner would result in a mentally advanced and physically strong child (these different data can be entered into a computer which will provide 'eugenic predictions'). As an illustration of the importance of the biological clock, the popular pamphlet *How to Give Birth to a Well-Behaved Baby* provides the example of a factory worker who married a peasant girl (both evidently of inferior stock by virtue of their low social station): their child entered Beijing University and later obtained a scholarship to study in the United States.[19] The choice of a season is also thought to be of considerable importance, since scientific research is said to demonstrate that children conceived by the end of autumn are intellectually more gifted than others: implicitly conceived in terms of *yin* and *yang* excesses, summer and winter are thought to lead to seasonal disorders which affect the health of pregnant women and can lead to foetal disorders.[20] These ideas are disseminated by popular medical literature, but they have achieved an even wider audience thanks to their often unscrupulous use by a variety of self-appointed experts in reproduction, all eager to sell their knowledge to an urban public only too willing to embrace products alleged

19 Liu Zhengxue, *Zenyang shengge guai wawa* (How to give birth to a well-behaved baby), Chengdu: Sichuan kexue jishu chubanshe, 1991, p. 7.
20 Lian Xiaohua, 'Zeshi shouyun hua yousheng' (Eugenics and the choice of the time for conception), *Renkou yu yousheng*, 1992, no. 3, p. 6.

to enhance the quality of offspring. These cultural and commercial trends combine to create fear and confusion, as is testified by complaints from social workers at genetic counselling units who report that some couples have chosen to have a child in disregard of local family planning regulations in order to comply with the requisites of their respective 'biological clocks':[21] even government circles thus seem at times outflanked by the powerful forces of social prejudice which they themselves have unleashed in their campaign for eugenics. These cultural representations of health and fitness shape actual reproductive behaviour in ways which sometimes contradict official policies.

BLOOD, GENES AND D.N.A.: THE INHERITANCE OF SOCIAL DEVIANCE

Health manuals provide useful information on a range of medical disorders and inherited diseases which can influence the health of future offspring. Medical knowledge, however, is also structured by a very normative approach to questions of reproductive health. As in traditional manuals of medicine, the choice of a fit partner is seen to be an essential requisite for the production of a viable baby. Moreover, health and ill-health are no longer visible qualities which the naked eye can discover. For example, heart disease, high blood pressure, diabetes, hepatitis and tuberculosis are 'hidden' ailments (*yinhuan*) which should be 'discovered' (*faxian*) in a premarital medical examination, since they can adversely affect foetal health if not cured before marriage. Other physical defects that influence the quality of offspring, such as

21 See for instance Yu Guanjian, 'Yousheng xuanchuan ying zhongshi kexuexing' (Eugenic propaganda should pay more attention to scientific credibility), *Renkou yu yousheng*, 1994, no. 2, p. 6 and Jiang Jianhong, '"Kexue youshengshu" bing bu kexue' ('Scientific art of eugenics' is not scientific at all), *Renkou yu yousheng*, 1990, no. 1, p. 7.

cryptorchism in the male and ovariopathy in the female, may remain concealed and have caused no ill-effect in other family members, yet they may be carried by pathogenic recessive genes. In medical language, a recessive gene is a 'hidden gene' (*yinxing jiyin*) ready to strike out and cripple descendants in the future. Notions of invisibility, concealment and latency are at the basis of an epistemology of 'discovery' in which medical experts alone are entitled to deliver a verdict of health. Genetic counselling is part of this process of medical assessment in which the criteria of health have become so elusive as virtually to designate each individual as potentially sick. As will be discussed in more detail below, all individuals are by definition the carriers of some 'gene' that might be identified as 'deleterious' or 'defective'. The frequent confusions made in health manuals between relatively benign disorders and grave inheritable diseases further contribute to an alarmist rhetoric of 'control' (*kongzhi*) and 'prevention' (*yufang*).

In manuals of medicine, normality and abnormality are expressed in medical terms, with the human body represented as a collection of bits and pieces which new technologies can gauge, measure and classify in ever more precise detail: reconfiguring a traditional link between health, balance and appearance, medical discourse parades sets of figures and statistics to estimate the degree of phenotypical conformity in an individual. The detection in a new-born baby of 'small ears', 'asymmetrical size of the ears', 'primitive shape of the ears', 'low-set ears', 'aurical tags', 'preaurical fistulas' or 'earlobe creases' thus warrants the birth being classified in medical textbooks as a 'defective birth'. Such level of precision is probably rarely used in actual medical practice, but it indicates how elusive ideals of normality have become as a much higher degree of specification is offered by new medical vocabularies. Specialist books based on empirical evidence obtained from hospitals also provide detailed lists of birth defects thought to have a hereditary basis, ranging from the 'simian crease' (*yuanxian*) to the 'single flexion

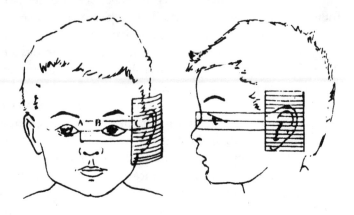

The measure of low-set ears.

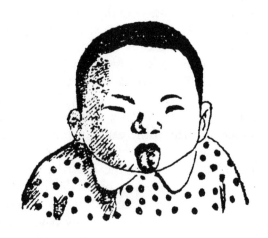

Congenital idiocy.

crease on fifth finger' and 'familial microcephalia' (*jiazuxing xiaotou*).[22]

A misleading sense of precision, based on mathematical statistics and sophisticated graphs, endows medical discourse with a tone of absolute authority as criteria of normality shift from individual cases to population trends. Providing medical élites and official circles with great powers of intervention, a focus on 'incidence', 'rates' and 'tendencies' underlines the pervasive nature of congenital disorders as curable conditions and infectious diseases are claimed to have been brought under control. A typical study observes that 23.44% of deaths of children under the age of fifteen in Beijing in 1974–6 were the result of a congenital disorder, while since the beginning of the 1970s 10% of infant mortality in Shanghai has been directly caused by foetal malformations.[23] The national consequences of dysgenic trends are described in stark terms: 'When a nation wants to stand on its own feet among the nations of the world, but does not have a robust physical constitution and fine intellectual resources, that goal may be difficult to achieve ... hence it is necessary to implement eugenics.'[24]

In the name of future generations and the physical wellbeing of the nation, health manuals enjoin young couples to seek eugenic advice in order to prevent the spread of 'hereditary diseases' (*yichuanbing*). Mental retardation, deafness, dwarfism and many other conditions are represented as 'hereditary diseases' to be brought under control. Following the guidelines of the Marriage Law of 1950 and 1980,[25] health manuals generally identify certain categories of people

22 Liu Chaoyu, *Yichuan yu chusheng quexian zonghezheng* (Heredity and malformations), Chengdu: Sichuan kexue jishu chubanshe, 1992.

23 Zhou Haobai, *Jitai zongheng tan* (Talks about malformations), Hangzhou: Jiangsu kexue jishu chubanshe, 1985, pp. 8–9.

24 Zhou, *Jitai*, p. 10.

25 See article 6 of the Marriage Law in *Population and Development Review* 7, no. 2 (1981).

as unfit for reproduction, in particular when both partners have a family history of 'hereditary diseases' or of intermarriage, or when both partners have been cured of a 'mental disease' (*jingshenbing*). In case only one partner has suffered from a psychotic disorder, special care should be taken after wedding (i.e. conception) and during pregnancy and breast-feeding to avoid a relapse. The popular booklet entitled *200 Questions about Foetal Education and Superior Birth*, in its fifth reprint two years after its publication in 1992 and selling more than 150,000 copies, further asserts that people afflicted with 'incurable' diseases, severe congenital malformations or hereditary diseases should be barred from marrying.[26]

Intelligence is also widely believed to be subject to the laws of inheritance, and a variety of authors underline that differences in the capacity to think, analyse and observe already exist at birth. Extensive research on 'retarded children' and 'child prodigies' by foreign experts is usually invoked to claim that education cannot substantially enhance intelligence and that eugenics is more effective in the 'production of gifted children'. 'Low intelligence' (*zhineng di*) and 'psychological disorders' (*jingshen fayu buliang*) are interpreted as polygenic traits that are genetically transmitted. Supported by investigations into family pedigrees, tables of statistics are meant to demonstrate that 55 to 60% of the children born to parents who both suffer from 'low intelligence' will be 'cretins' (*daizi*), the remaining 40% also being below par.[27] 'Superior intelligence [*shangzhi*] and inferior stupidity [*xiayu*] cannot be changed,' the classics of Confucianism claimed long ago.[28] Premier Li Peng has put it

26 Luo Hong and Jiang Chaoguang, *Taijiao yu yousheng 200 wen* (200 questions about foetal education and superior birth), Beijing: Jindun chubanshe, 1992 (5th repr. 1994), pp. 28–31.

27 Zhou Haobai, *Jitai zongheng tan* (Talks about malformations), Hangzhou: Jiangsu kexue jishu chubanshe, 1985, p. 319.

28 *Lunyu* (Analects), *Yanghuo*, 17:3.

in less ambivalent terms in a public statement: 'Idiots breed idiots'.[29]

Just as folk notions represent madness as a somatic defect running in family lines, so medical discourse underlines the genetic basis of mental disease, which it interprets as an organic lesion, a blot on the brain or a hereditary taint that is almost incurable. As one popular booklet on family planning put it, 'There are many types of mental disease, such as schizophrenia, manic-depressive psychosis and paranoia, and all have a genetic basis. The rate of occurrence among relatives of sufferers of mental disease is significantly higher in comparison to the average, and the results of research demonstrate that when both parents suffer from mental disease, 40% of their offspring will also be sufferers. If one side is affected by mental disease, 2–4% of their children will be sufferers. Hence people who suffer from mental disease should not marry among themselves, since they are not only unable to live independently, but the risk of them giving birth to offspring with mental disease is also great. [...] No matter whether one or both parents suffer from mental disease, they should neither marry nor reproduce when the disease is active.'[30] If medical circles advocate a strict ban on the reproduction of those deemed 'mad',[31] some psychiatrists in the PRC have themselves been very concerned with the genetics of 'schizophrenia', and a few have recommended and enforced a eugenic policy of compulsory sterilisation well before the enactment of the 1995 Eugenics Law.[32]

Consanguineous marriages, in which genetically dominant diseases are said to occur in disproportionately high

---

29 Nicolas D. Kristof, 'Parts of China forcibly sterilizing the retarded who wish to marry', *New York Times*, 15 August 1991, p. 1.

30 Weng, *Jihua shengyu*, p. 101.

31 For instance Hu Weiqin, 'Jingshen bingren de hunyin wenti' (The question of marriage for mentally sick people), *Renkou yu yousheng*, 1988, no. 1, p. 11.

32 Veronica Pearson, 'Population policy and eugenics in China', *British Journal of Psychiatry*, 1995, 167, p. 3; see also Veronica Pearson, *Mental health care in China: State policies, professional services and family responsibilities*, London: Gaskell, 1995.

numbers, are singled out for special opprobrium: emblematic of benighted rural practices to be swept away by medical enlightenment in the name of collective health, they are claimed to be the main factor responsible for mental retardation and other 'genetic' conditions in the countryside. Repeated *ad nauseam* in popular health manuals and corroborated by a spate of professional opinions in specialised journals, the emphasis on the genetic basis of mental retardation and the medical dangers of inbreeding dominate eugenic discourse. In a medical language of 'hidden defects' and 'genetic loads' – not without resonance to the Buddhist karma – the responsibility of each and every individual in the choice of a marital partner is stressed:

> The closer the blood relationship, the higher the chance of encounter between deleterious genes, hence the bigger the probability of genetic diseases among progeny. According to statistics, the incidence of a genetically transmitted disease is 150 times higher in progeny of a consanguineous couple than in a normal couple. Mainly because of our country's exceedingly narrow marriage circle, we have more than 10 million congenitally handicapped people, approximately 20% of the total of handicapped people. [...] Inbreeding causes disadvantageous recessive genes to become dominant. Under the stimulation of a harmful factor, inbreeding may cause some hidden defective genes to change into active and apparent ones. Among a group of healthy people, each person is also the carrier of about five to six harmful genes, which also means that their children have a chance to suffer from a genetically transmitted disease: this is the genetic load. This genetic load becomes actual through inbreeding, hence the unhealthy genes of our country's gene pool incessantly increase. Because previously we did not pay sufficient attention to genetics, the population of our country has 25 to 30% of people who have some sort of hereditary disease. This signifies that the quality of our

future generations is seriously endangered, a trend which we can decidedly not allow to develop any further. Moreover, inbreeding lowers the intelligence quotient of progeny.[33]

As the 'gene pool' gradually becomes a metaphor for the social field, statistical tables are provided to demonstrate the inevitability of mental retardation and physical weakness in offspring of marriages between close relatives. Reports from hospitals are invoked to demonstrate how close relatives produce feeble-minded offspring: 'One famous professor in Beijing and his wife were both healthy in body and mind but gave birth to three retarded daughters. When their genes were checked, it appeared that they were close cousins. These retarded children were able to survive thanks to the conditions created by civilised society, but if they were allowed to marry in turn, the consequences would be even worse. In one place, a retarded couple gave birth to a series of six retarded children.'[34] In most modernising nations, eugenic arguments have usually targeted consanguinity, because of the belief that it is conducive to a biologically impoverished and medically dangerous line of descent. Although historians of medicine have generally taken 'inbreeding' as an objective given, an entire cluster of cultural and social values, rather than straightforward factual knowledge, has clearly endowed the notion of consanguinity with a rich layer of different meanings. Consanguinity is closely linked to older ideas of patrilineality, and represents isolation in a world of movement, symbolises a closed and self-contained localism in an age of open and interdependent globalism, and backward rural ways in opposition to the modern city. An inbreeding

33 Zhu Hong, 'Lianyin fanwei yu renkou suzhi' (The scope of marriage and population quality), *Zhong Gong Zhejiang Shengwei Dangxiao* (Communist Party of China's Zhejiang Provincial Party Committee School), March 1990, pp. 29–35, reprinted in *Renkouxue* (Demographic studies), 1990, no. 5, pp. 96–100.
34 Zhao Gongmin, *Yichuanxue yu shehui* (Genetics and society), Shenyang: Liaoning renmin chubanshe, 1986, p. 210.

village is seen as a pocket of resistance against the forces of modernity, and thus is necessarily marked out for special attention in the cultural landscape of almost every modernising country. In their scientisation of the incest taboo, medical ideas against 'inbreeding' often say more about social values than about genetic facts. Just as the medical arguments occasionally invoked against 'miscegenation' between imagined 'races' determine the outer limits of a social field in which it is morally acceptable to form a relationship, so the notion of 'consanguinity' identifies the inner limits of admissible reproductive behaviour. It defines the minimum level of participation of the individual in the social field and fixes a threshold of tolerance below which intimate behaviour is seen to be morally corrupt and biologically degenerative. Legitimising the reach of the government into families and lineages, it endows society with unprecedented powers of intervention and regulation into the personal lives of individuals in the name of public health.

'Peasants' and 'minorities' are the two most important social groups which have been singled out for medical opprobrium, as if their political and economic marginalisation is somehow justified by a deeper genetic liminality: it is claimed in numerous medical studies that inbreeding has wrought havoc on these more 'feudal' (fengjian) and 'backward' (luohou) communities. Frequent studies on 'intermarriage' appear in the learned journals of genetics and anthropology, pointing both to their cultural backwardness and their genetic inferiority. To take a single example among the dozens to be found in these journals, one team surveyed five 'minority' groups in Xinjiang and found that consanguineous marriages had significantly increased among the Hui and the Uyghur, leading to a variety of genetic diseases.[35] Some of these studies have been carried out by

35 Ai Qionghua *et al.*, 'Xinjiang Yili wuge shaoshu minzu de jinqin jiehun' (Consanguineous marriages among five minority nationalities in Yili, Xinjiang), *Renleixue xuebao*, 1985, no. 3, pp. 242–9.

'minority' scientists. For instance, Abdullah Bake revealed
that the Uyghur of Turpan suffer from dangerously high
rates of inbreeding ranging from 16.5 to 21.7%, and called
for increased government intervention in the control of
reproduction.[36] While minority groups no doubt suffer from
a variety of diseases, the belief that their social and economic
problems are caused by inbreeding is often no more than a
scientised version of Han prejudice against Hui endogamic
practices.[37]

Identifying the 'peasants' as the core of dysgenic tendencies, the journal *Population and Eugenics*, published for a popular audience by the Population Research Centre of
Zhejiang Medical College in Hangzhou, deplores the
increasing number of 'sub-products' (*cipin*) and 'reject products' (*feipin*) born every year: knowledge of eugenics among
peasants is very poor, they have 'ugly habits' (*chengui louxi*),
and they frequently intermarry or reproduce outside the
marital bond.[38] Even the newly-rich villages are alleged to
have a high percentage of retardation, 80% of which is
described as 'light retardation' (*qingdu zhiruo*). Although this
is explained by consanguineous marriages, the second major
factor is said to be the life-style of these *nouveau riche* peasants, who 'don't read books, don't read newspapers, lead an
unhealthy lifestyle, drink alcohol, smoke cigarettes, gamble
and whore, and even take concubines and drugs, thus directly endangering the health of the next generation, engender-

---

36 Abudula Bakhy, 'Tulufan shijiaoqu Weiwuerzu de jinqin jiehunlü ji yichuanxue xiaoying' (Rates of inbreeding and their genetic effects in Uyghurs of the
suburbs of Turpan), *Yichuan*, 1996, no. 3, pp. 252–3; some aspects of genetic
research on minorities are analysed in Frank Dikötter, 'Reading the body:
Genetic knowledge and social marginalisation in the PRC', *China Information*,
12, no. 4 (Spring 1998).
37 Dru C. Gladney, *Muslim Chinese: Ethnic nationalism in the People's Republic*,
Cambridge, MA: Harvard University Press, 1996, pp. 252–8.
38 'Tigao renkou suzhi de guanjian zai nongcun' (The key to improving the
quality of the population lies in the countryside), *Renkou yu yousheng*, 1993,
no. 1, pp. 24–5.

ing one batch after the other of retarded children.'[39] Because
illiterates and half-literates reproduced themselves so quickly
in the countryside, natural selection laws in which 'the superior win and the inferior lose' (*yousheng liebai*) were replaced
by a more worrying trend of 'the inferior win and the superior lose' (*liesheng youbai*).[40]

'The higher the level of education, the lower the number
of children' concludes a more detailed study of genetic
trends in Fujian province, where in strict numerical terms
the least gifted members of society are shown to contribute
seventy-five times more children than intellectuals: the article proposes the immediate targeting of genetic diseases and
inbreeding in the countryside.[41] Wang Ruizi, vice-director
of a demography centre in Hangzhou, noting how vagrants
block traffic in cities and indulge in criminal activities, similarly points out that the great majority of handicapped people are to be found in the countryside.[42] In the early 1990s,
concern over the differential birthrate between urbanites,
who were seen as embodying the more gifted parts of the
population, and peasants, who were portrayed as a demographic wasteland of retardant and mutants, prompted
Population and Eugenics to advocate a eugenic policy similar
to that enacted in Singapore: genetically fitter elements
should be encouraged to have more than one child while
massive disincentives would contribute to checking dysgenic

39 Tao Kan, 'Fushu diqu yuanhe ruozhi ertong yuelai yueduo' (Why retarded children are on the increase in rich and populous regions), *Renkou yu yousheng*, 1996, no. 4, p. 3.
40 Wang Ruogu, 'Wen Xinjiapo xin renkou zhengce you gan' (The population policy in Singapore), *Renkou yu yousheng*, 1992, no. 4, p. 26.
41 Chen Yandong, 'Tigao renkou suzhi dui kongzhi renkou shuliang de zhanlüe yiyi' (The strategic meaning of improving the quality of the population versus limiting the quantity of the population), *Renkou yu yousheng*, 1991, no. 1, pp. 18–19.
42 Wang Ruizi, 'Zhongguo renkou wenti de zhongdian zai nongcun' (The core of demographic problems is in the countryside), *Renkou yu yousheng*, 1991, no. 2, pp. 3–4.

trends in the countryside. Enthusiastic responses from readers have been published in support of these views.[43]

While such reactions should be taken with a grain of salt in a one-party state where the press is presumed to offer a close reflection of official policies, there is mounting evidence that educated people resent the existing disparities between cities and countryside in the implementation of the one-child programme. Eugenic arguments are voiced against population policies that are seen as contributing to a differential growth-rate between the more gifted members of the urban population and the vast hordes of dysgenic elements represented by migrants, 'peasants' and paupers. Under pressure from the medical experts and family planners who present such ideas in the guise of 'science', the government is alleged to have moved in 1996 towards a policy of encouraging urban dwellers and educated people to have more babies while discouraging 'peasants' from doing so, on the grounds that 'quality stock' is indispensable to China's modernisation. The government would have accepted the recommendation of a task force that parents likely to produce more intelligent children be eugenically selected.[44]

As the one-child policy has created a social environment in which parents themselves are keen to engender 'superior' offspring, some publications have moved beyond the specification of what is seen to constitute medical health towards the identification of what is thought to be socially desirable. Reinforcing folk notions which associate physical stature with intelligence, popular booklets written in the name of medical science provide a panoply of means to increase one's height.[45] For Dai Zhi, author of a booklet

43 See for instance the letter published in *Renkou yu yousheng*, 1993, no. 5, p. 45.
44 "More babies move" for China's well-educated', *Straits Times*, 29 Aug. 1996.
45 Similar ideas had already appeared in republican China. In a popular introduction to the 'science of body measurements', Jiang Xiangqing (1899–1981) established that a strong correlation between height and intelligence was at the basis of 'race', sex and class differences. Jiang Xiangqing, who was to become deputy president of the Shanghai Sports Training School in communist China, noted

entitled *The Most Recent Science and Technology for Increasing Body Height*, 'Short bodies often have a poor quality such as weak physical strength and an inferior intelligence.'[46] Written as a contribution to the increase of the 'Chinese nation's height', the book also exposes eugenic means of producing bigger bodies and encourages young people to choose tall marriage partners, since height is a hereditary feature which can be passed on to future generations.

'SUPERIOR BIRTHS': THE SCIENCE OF FOETAL EDUCATION

Folk notions of maternal influence, which have a long pedigree in both popular and élite culture, are given the seal of approval by medical experts. Consolidating a somatising approach, scientific studies are conducted to adduce evidence for the existence of a strong link between the emotions of the mother and the development of the foetus. After an earthquake ravaged the city of Tangshan in July 1976 (this natural catastrophe was popularly interpreted as a celestial portent for an imminent dynastic collapse, which was confirmed by the death of chairman Mao less than two months later), researcher Li Yurong carried out a comparison between 206 children born to women who were pregnant during the disaster and 144 children from regions where no earthquake had occurred. Intelligence tests showed that the earthquake group of children had an average IQ of 86.43

---

that the upper classes were generally taller than the lower classes and expressed this relationship in a concise sentence: 'the more stupid, the smaller'; see Jiang Xiangqing, *Renti celiangxue* (The science of body measurements), Shanghai: Qinfen shuju, 1935, pp. 97–8.

46 Dai Zhi, *Renti zenggao de zuixin kexue jishu* (The newest technology to increase body height), Beijing: Zhongguo yiyao keji chubanshe, 1993, pp. 74–83 and 133–6; see also Liao Zhifang and Zhong Xin, *Renti zenggao de mijue* (Secrets to increase body height), Guangxi kexue jishu chubanshe, 1991.

compared to 91.95 in the second group: these results were thought to illustrate how a natural disaster could upset the emotional economy of pregnant women, influencing in turn the development of the foetus's nervous system.[47]

Even minor emotional shocks are said to present a threat to foetal health, as popular culture and medical discourse converge in the idea that the moral character and emotional disposition of a pregnant woman have a direct relationship with birth defects. Thus, negative emotions can considerably intensify the activity of the vegetative nervous system and liberate harmful particles which affect the development of the foetus, which is particularly sensitive during the first three months of pregnancy.[48] Another pamphlet of advice on how to obtain eugenically meritorious offspring insists on the devastating consequences of strong emotions – anxiety, melancholy, rage – which prevent the correct functioning of superior nervous activity (the author uses Pavlovian vocabulary) of the cerebral cortex: it leads to a harelip or a cleft palate, among other malformations.[49] The hugely successful primer entitled *Three Hundred Questions on Health during Pregnancy*, of which almost half a million copies were printed, also explains that anxiety and fear can stimulate the production of excessive quantities of adrenocortical hormones, so inducing physical abnormalities in the foetus.[50] Even a detailed and comprehensive treatise on obstetrics designed for the professionals, written by a medical team of Zhejiang province, underlines the need for 'mental hygiene' (*xinli weisheng*), including a positive mood, optimistic outlook and

47 Liu Zhengxue, *Zenyang shengge guai wawa* (How to give birth to a well-behaved baby), Chengdu: Sichuan kexue jishu chubanshe, 1991, p. 63.

48 Yang Xiuting *et al.* (eds), *Taijiao, weiyang, baojian* (Foetal education, child feeding and health protection), Harbin: Heilongjiang jiaoyu chubanshe, 1988, p. 3.

49 Luo Hong and Jiang Chaoguang, *Taijiao yu yousheng 200 wen* (200 questions about foetal education and superior birth), Beijing: Jindun chubanshe, 1992 (5th repr. 1994), pp. 128–9.

50 Xing Shumin, *Yunchanfu baojian 300 wen* (Three hundred questions on health during pregnancy), Beijing: Jindun chubanshe, 1991 (10th repr. 1994), pp. 54–5.

a harmonious family life, in order to exert a positive influence on the development of the foetus.[51] Emotions can induce biochemical changes in the body, and ultrasounds demonstrate that the foetus responds to emotional shocks. A cleft palate is interpreted as a consequence of emotional instability during pregnancy, but a minor one since severe disruption can even cause foetal death. On the other hand, a positive environment can enhance the mental capacity and physical appearance of the foetus. For instance, reading books that are 'healthy and morally edifying' (*jiankang youyi*) can help to create an ideal atmosphere for pregnant women; and by analogy, socially deviant types of literature may lead to biologically disordered offspring. None of these ideas concerning prenatal health are specifically eugenist, and many of them can be found in the medical literature of developed countries. However, it is important not too dismiss such ideas as superstitious or even ridiculous, but to underline how advice on reproductive health is offered within a broadly eugenist framework with strong normative values. Moreover, medical discourse is governed by representations of female vulnerability and assigns the principal responsibility over reproduction to women.

In its representation of gender distinctions, which are seen as biologically determined structures naturally complementing each other, medical discourse also attributes duties to the male partner. As in late imperial China, the father's contribution is believed to lie in the quality of his sperm. A direct relationship is constructed by analogy between physical health and seminal strength. Because their state of mind directly affects their generative power, both partners should be in high spirits at the moment of conception: 'Low morale, mental nervousness and difficult living conditions are not conducive to the bearing of high-quality offspring.'[52]

---

51 Wang Man *et al.* (eds), *Shiyong fuchanke shouce* (Handbook of applied obstetrics), Zhejiang kexue jishu chubanshe, 1989.
52 Fang and Hou, *Youshengxue*, p. 303.

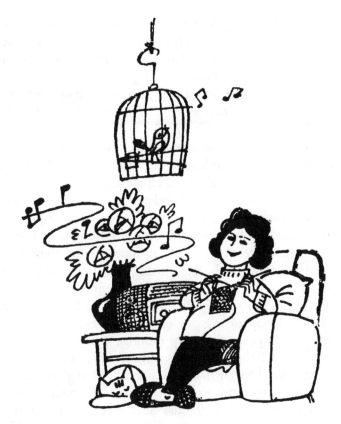

A joyful outlook during pregnancy.

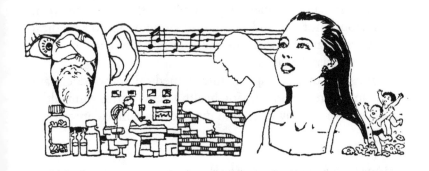

Foetal education.

Many examples of parental responsibility over foetal health are given by popular medical handbooks. In one example, a child was born with malformations that affected almost every part of the body, including an imperforate anus, supernumerary fingers, absence of reproductive organs and major damage to the internal organs. The mother worked as a sewing-machine operator and the father was an electrician. Both enjoyed good health and their families had no history of inherited diseases, although the father was a heavy smoker and frequently drank alcohol. However, the couple already had a bright young son and did not wish to have a second child, so much so that when the mother became pregnant, she hid her condition and did not consult a doctor right up till the time of delivery: 'One can imagine her dodging and anxious psychological state during her pregnancy, which must have caused havoc to the functioning of the internal secretions, so influencing the development of the foetus and in particular obstructing the 'process of moulding the form' [*suzao chengxing*] in the early months, adding to the harm caused by the father's smoking and drinking. This is precisely what caused foetal malformations.'[53] Mental convulsions are claimed somehow to have imprinted themselves on the distorted body of the foetus. Similar examples stress the importance of human agency and locate the causes of illness in the behaviour of both parents. They are part of a mode of causality which explains the universe in terms of individual behaviour and human responsibility: the link between behaviour, morality and health is reconfigured into a medical discourse that represents the monster as a biological retribution for social deviation.

In its pursuit of a eugenic future, medical knowledge maps out an entire geography of health, demarcating unhealthy places from healthy ones, and discovering sanitary interstices

---

53 Na Li, *Taijiao fangfa* (Methods of foetal education), Beijing: Zhongyang minzu xueyuan chubanshe, 1988, pp. 49–50.

within the baneful texture spun by modernity: pregnant women should visit parks, gardens, beaches and other uncontaminated spaces where nature can be admired and 'beautiful scenery' (*meili fengguang*) can exert its beneficial influence on the foetus.[54] A regulated lifestyle with clear rules (*you guilü de shenghuo*) will engender a disciplined child, and the pregnant mother should follow a strict routine to instil a sense of measure into the foetus. Classical music, symbolising ordered harmony, can help to convey a notion of balance, whereas popular music performed by socially deviant categories of people is thought to transmit deviance, since rock and roll music can bring about negative reactions in the foetus.

Medical discourse establishes a strict delineation between 'causes' and 'effects' in a holistic approach which represents embryological life as an indissoluble whole of a higher human collectivity. Because society is thought to influence and shape its development, marking the foetus with its signature even before it can breathe, these external forces should be harnessed and guided in a eugenic direction. Typical of this vision of eugenic improvement is the invention in 1990 by Tu Xing, a gynaecological specialist, of a 'microphone for foetal education' (*taijiao huatong*), to be placed on the mother's belly to transmit educational material such as classical music, language lessons, traditional poetry and moral tales that will contribute to building the character and developing the intelligence of the future child (the product has received a patent). A research team of doctors, psychologists and electricians in Tianjin, has gone further; in 1990 it developed a 'foetal education multi-functional electrical instrument' (*duo dianzi taijiao yi*) capable of transmitting educational material at regular intervals to the foetus; it can also transform the real voices of outsiders into a melodious tone that is pleasant for

---

54 Beijing fuchan yiyuan (eds), *Fuchan ji ying'er de yingyang yu baojian* (Health protection and nutrition for pregnant women and infants), Beijing: Zhongguo shangye chubanshe, 1990, p. 21.

the foetus to listen to.[55] Harmonious melodies and balanced rhythms are scientifically designed to appeal to the undeveloped central nervous system of the foetus. Similar instruments, of course, have also appeared on the market in developed countries, including Britain and the United States, although they are not sold as part of a wider eugenic programme. While such commercial products might appeal to any parent concerned with the healthy development of the foetus, the existing population policies and health programmes have endowed them with a more eugenic meaning which is unique to the PRC. As has already been noted in this chapter, such products also play on the belief in a strong retributive link between the behaviour of the parents and the quality of their offspring.

Tapes to be played for the foetus have also been developed and marketed in huge quantities in China, from children's songs to lessons in the correct pronunciation of Mandarin. Some of these tapes have been designed and produced by the Chinese Medical Association. The association's first tape, designed by a team of psychologists and released on the market in 1985, achieved sales of more than 300,000 by the summer of 1988. Some of its hits include 'Mama and me together', 'I want to speak with mama' and 'Mama's honey-sweet breasts'. The use of these new educational methods is not confined to private individuals; they have also been enthusiastically adopted by some birth planning institutions. The Foetal Education Office of the Fengfu Cigarette Factory Birth Planning Clinic (sic) in Anhui Province, to take but one example, proudly announced its adoption of electrical devices for the education of foetuses aged more than five months in 1995.[56] Computers and genetics are the two hobby-horses of China before the millennium, and it is

55 An Hao and Kang Jindong, *Taijiao yu'er zhidao* (Guide to foetal education), Tianjin: Nankai daxue chubanshe, 1992, pp. 94–5.
56 Shen Huiyun, 'Wo chang de "taijiao" shi' (Our factory's 'foetal education' office), *Renkou yu yousheng*, 1995, no. 47, p. 9.

not surprising that they meet in the development of computer software concerned with hereditary diseases. Designed by the Daping Hospital in Sichuan province, it contains all the medical knowledge available for the diagnosis and prevention of more than 2,000 genetic defects, and is claimed to be able to 'predict whether parents with congenital defects will have healthy children'.[57]

The recent progress in reproductive technologies and genetic engineering is also seen as a helpful step forward towards implementation of positive eugenics in order to improve the genetic quality of mankind and to produce ideal babies. Calls for positive eugenics, designed to make 'superior' people breed 'superior' offspring, occasionally appear in both popular and specialised literature. Zhu Hong, a party member at the Zhejiang Provincial Party Committee School, upholds such a view: 'There is a clause allowing the parents of a first child who is handicapped to bear a second child: this should be replaced by a clause forbidding parents of a first child who has a hereditary handicap to bear a second child. In the mean time, some people distantly related by blood with high intelligence quotients, like outstanding scientists, mathematicians, writers, musicians, top sportsmen and others, should be encouraged to have a second child within the family plan.'[58] Embryo transplants, artificial insemination, external fertilisation and test-tube babies are often mentioned as useful medical technologies that might project mankind into a eugenic future.[59] The sperm bank funded by the American millionaire Robert K. Graham in 1971, reserved exclusively for donations of sperm from Nobel laureates and located today in Escondido, California, under the name of Repository for Germinal Choice, is welcomed as a major

57 'Software developed for diagnosing hereditary diseases', SWB, 15 February 1995, FEW/0371/WG/11.
58 Zhu, 'Lianyin fanwei', pp. 96–100.
59 See for instance Liu Qingxian, 'Kua shiji de shengzhi geming' (A reproductive revolution which straddles the next century), Yixue yu zhexue, 1994, no. 4, pp. 33–4.

breakthrough in the genetic control of mankind. When calls are made for the extensive use of sperm banks, there is often insistence on strict medical checking of potential sperm donors, including a genetic profile as well as an intelligence test. In an effort to catch up with these developments abroad, the Hunan hospital has been hailed as the first hospital in China to have a sperm bank: it started artificially inseminating women in the early 1980s.

Births of test-tube babies, first successfully achieved in England in 1978, have also been announced in China since March 1988. According to one popular booklet on foetal education and eugenics, those chosen to contribute sperm and eggs for the production of test-tube babies should have 'distinctively superior genes' as well as 'excellent intellectual abilities and physical appearance'.[60] One of the few objections to the widespread production of test-tube babies is that anonymous donors might inadvertently turn out to be close relatives, thereby increasing the rate of inbreeding. An optimistic author envisages that this process — the large-scale selection of donors whose germ-cells are proved to be of superior quality, their storage into a 'Eugenics Bank Centre', and their use to propagate 'superior bodies' — will have become a genuine possibility by the year 2015.[61] Even the extreme expedient of engineering a new race of humanoids, useful for both military and civil purposes (among their prospective tasks would be the cleaning up of nuclear waste), has been envisaged, although such views seem not to have a serious following. Recalling experiments allegedly conducted up till 1966 in Liaoning province, in which a female chimpanzee was artificially inseminated with human semen so as to engender a new cross between humans and apes for

60 Fang Fang, *Yousheng yu youyu* (Eugenics and quality childbirth), Beijing: Renmin chubanshe, 1991, pp. 25–8.
61 Qu Jianding, 'Cong ziran xuanze dao rengong xuanze: tan renkou shenti suzhi he yichuan jiyin' (From natural selection to artificial selection: About inherited genes and the physical quality of the population), repr. in *Renkouxue*, 1987, no. 2, pp. 76–8.

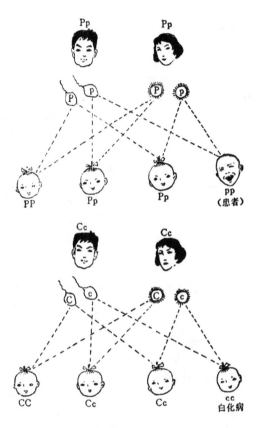

The genetics of albinism.

use in the army, such endeavours are condemned as unethical and utopian (the chimpanzee was three months pregnant at the start of the Cultural Revolution and reportedly died before it could give birth).[62]

The cloning of human germ cells, a reproductive technology that would involve neither sperm nor egg, is also discussed as a future possibility in the arsenal of eugenic measures.[63] Although eugenic discourse in itself does not

-62 Huang Jianmin, 'Fandui zaochu xin renzhong' (Against the making of a new race), *Jiankang shijie*, 1996, no. 6, pp. 38–9.
63 Qu, 'Cong ziran xuanze', pp. 76–8.

inevitably entail the promotion of racial categories of analysis, since it focuses on the genetic fitness of individuals within a country rather than as between population groups defined as 'races', some publications in demography nonetheless advance claims about the 'biological fitness' of the nation and herald the next century as an era to be dominated by 'biological competition' between the 'white race' and the 'yellow race'.[64] The mastery of reproductive technologies and genetic engineering is seen as being crucial in this future battle of the genes, and the government has given much support to medical research in human genetics. A research team was even set up in November 1993 to isolate the quintessentially 'Chinese genes' of the genetic code of human DNA.[65]

LIMINAL FIGURES: THE MEDICAL SEMIOLOGY OF MONSTERS

Since the beginning of the 1980s, public health pamphlets and travelling exhibitions graphically exhibit the commonest birth defects, including photographs of malformed foetuses.[66] Such exhibits usually explain laws of inheritance in human beings, depicting how a 'normal' parent crossed with an 'abnormal' one may still produce an 'abnormal' child. Framed by an image or bottled in a jar, the body of the mon-

64 See for instance Wang Ruiduo, 'Jiantan renkou zhiliang yu shehui fazhan de guanxi' (Brief discussion about the relationship between population quality and social development), *Renkouxue*, 1987, no. 1, p. 110.
65 Lincoln Kaye, 'Quality control: Eugenics bill defended against Western critics', *Far Eastern Economic Review*, 13 January 1994, p. 22.
66 In one of the worst examples of this type of didactic literature, a popular journal on eugenics illustrated the 'bitter wine fermented by opposing eugenics' with gross photographs of two lovers with visible deformities in the limbs and their severely deformed baby, who was presumed to be the result of their secret cohabitation; see Xiao Hua, 'Jixing hunyin jixing er' (Freak marriage leads to freak child); *Renkou yu yousheng*, 1992, no. 2, p. 10; many similar articles and broadsheets have been published since the end of the 1980s.

ster is a culturally constructed object which symbolically represents the physical retribution of unregulated reproduction. In the PRC, an entire range of different meanings are ascribed to 'monsters', which represent almost anything from a pregnant women's failure to control her emotions to modern man's alienation from a polluted environment.

While most of the medical literature is concerned with common disabilities and relatively widespread birth defects, the more extraordinary phenomena of 'monsters' have also become a popular topic for public entertainment. Wild men and bearded women, giants and dwarfs, hermaphrodites, conjoined twins and three-legged humans: an entire range of liminal figures occupy a prominent position in a cultural field structured by a fascination with the abnormal. In a distant echo of the imperial canon of prodigies, popular booklets on freaks cater to the general public's craving for the strange and weird.[67] Written under the guise of medical science, but reminiscent in its presentation of late imperial literary sketches (*biji*) of strange events, the *Record of fantastic stories about the human body* (1989) for instance provides the reader with detailed anecdotes ranging from a primitive race of green people in the dark forests of Africa to a wild girl aged seven brought up by monkeys. Evoking the formal categories of medical science, congenital malformations figure prominently in the sections on anatomy and physiology: a limbless infant, a two-headed baby, a pregnant boy, a girl without a chest, a man with two tongues, a women with eight breasts, a blue-skinned tribe and many other freaks are all given pride of place in this publication compiled by a team of the Shaanxi Hospital of Chinese Medicine.[68]

'Hairy children' in particular became objects of wonder during the 1980s. Constructed as a medical category with

67 For example Wang Yijiong, *Renti zhi mi* (Mysteries of the human body), Shanghai: Wenhui chubanshe, 1988.
68 Sun Puquan, *Renti qiwen lu* (Record of fantastic stories about the human body), Zhengzhou: Tianze chubanshe, 1989.

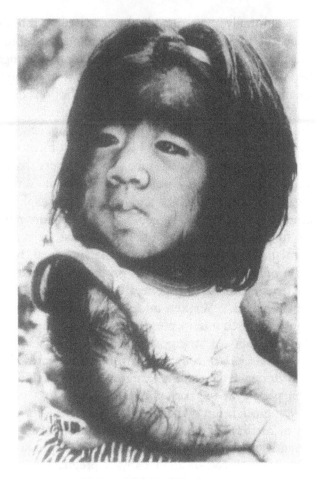

Hairy child Yu Zhenhuan.

finite borders, 'hairy people' (*maoren*) became the exclusive object of investigation of a special unit set up by the department of biology of Liaoning University in 1978. The unit published the results of its investigation with a collection of photographs of thirty-two cases from China four years later.[69] Aptly illustrating the resilience of recapitulation theo-

---

69 Liu Mingyu *et al.* (eds), *Zhongguo maoren* (Hairy men of China), Shenyang: Liaoning kexue jishu chubanshe, 1982.

ry in China, the first sentence of the book concisely summarised the conclusion reached by the team: 'Hairy people are racial atavisms'. The greater part of the book focused on Yu Zhenhuan, an astonishing case of hypertrichosis whose development had been closely charted by the Liaoning University team (see illustration opposite). Covered with long hair on most parts of the body, Yu Zhenhuan was taken as the most pristine example of a 'racial reversion'. Three other cases of hairy children, born in the same year as Yu Zhenhuan, were also brought to the attention of the public. Similar to explanations popular in Europe during the 1920s, the hereditary aspects of hypertrichosis were highlighted by the pedigree of four families in which aberrant hair growth had occurred over two to three generations. If the myth of racial atavism dated from the late nineteenth century, the only scientific reference of the authors was a sentence in Charles Darwin's *Descent of Man*: 'Three or four cases have been recorded of persons born with their whole bodies and faces thickly covered with fine long hairs; and this strange condition is strongly inherited and is correlated with an abnormal condition of the teeth.' The fear of dissolution and the desire to control was most evident in the suggestion that 'positive and effective measures' be implemented to prevent the spread of hypertrichosis to the rest of the population. Yu Zhenhuan rapidly became a popular marvel: news on television, reports in the official press, feature articles in more popular magazines brought the general public images of the 'hairy child'. A widely distributed *Mysteries of the human body* (1989), to take but one instance, had an entire paragraph devoted to 'hairy people' and reported the story of Yu Zhenhuan in compelling detail.[70]

---

70 Zou Guangzhong, *Renti zhi mi* (Mysteries of the human body), Beijing: Xinhua chubanshe, 1989, pp. 53–6.

EUGENIC LAWS AND REPRODUCTIVE HEALTH

Not without resemblance to Confucian notions of self-cultivation and self-restraint, the mass education campaigns in
reproductive health and the medical knowledge dispensed to
prospective parents are meant to ensure the participation of
each individual in the regeneration of the nation. Where
couples fail to reproduce eugenically, the state can intervene
in the name of collective health. Numerous publications
advocate the elimination *in utero* of foetuses defined as
'defective'. According to Zhou Xiaozheng, affiliated with
the Population Research Centre of Beijing University, widespread prenatal testing should warrant the detection of
'monsters' (*jixing'er*) at an early stage of pregnancy, while the
abortion of foetuses with minor defects such as a harelip or
supernumerary fingers could take place between the eighteenth and the twentieth week.[71] The moral value and economic meaning of euthanasia have been regularly underlined
in journals on demography and medical ethics at least since
1990, while the elimination of new-born infants with severe
malformations is rarely seen to pose any particular ethical
problems.[72] Professor Zhao Gongmin, a Fudan University
graduate in biology with a specialisation in genetics and a
Fellow of the Chinese Academy of Social Science, considers
the social benefits of euthanasia to outweigh any moral considerations: 'As to those already born and afflicted with
severe inherited malformations, such as cretins with a
stretched tongue (*shenshe chidai*, children with Down's syn-

71 Zhou Xiaozheng, 'Ershiyi shiji de Zhongguo renkou yu yousheng' (The
Chinese population and eugenics in the twenty-first century), *Renkouxue*, 1988,
no. 4, p. 83.
72 Yuan Huarong, 'Lun yousi de shehui jingji yiyi he daode jiazhi' (About the
social and economic meaning of euthanasia and its moral value), *Renkou yanjiu*,
1990, no. 4; on the debates around the mercy-killing of neonates and terminally-
ill patients, see Frank Dikötter, 'Death by design: Euthanasia in China' (forthcoming).

drome) or babies suffering from hydrocephalus, their intelligence is very low and even if they can survive, they will never be able to work and live independently, giving their families endless misfortunes, increasing the burden on society and adversely influencing the quality of the population. Painless euthanasia at the moment that such babies appear to the world, it should be said, is a eugenic measure that will benefit the country and the people.'[73]

In an article published in the respected *Sociological Research* and reprinted in the April 1991 issue of *Demography*, Mu Guangzong, a lecturer at the Population Studies Centre of the People's University and one of the most vocal proponents of euthanasia, proposes a sociological definition of medical death called 'zero worth' (*ling suzhi*): individuals are intrinsic parts of a larger collectivity, and their worth is defined by the contribution they can make to society. As 'inferior births' have 'zero worth' and make no such contribution, society has the right medically to eliminate them. According to Mu Guangzong, the warning of the great Victorian scientist T.H. Huxley should be heeded: if the quality of life is not strictly controlled, bad genetic mutations will accumulate and mankind will head towards suicide.[74]

Euthanasia is seen as a means to achieve a 'scientific humanism' (*kexue rendaozhuyi*) that protects society against 'counter-selective' forces (*ni taotai*) represented by disabled infants. Writing five years before the 1996 controversy of the 'dying rooms', in which a 'Channel Four' documentary on the British television channel claimed that certain orphanages deliberately starved some abandoned children to death, Mu deplores the 'zero worth' of orphans with disabilities who survive in state welfare institutions: just as eugenics prevents

73 Zhao, *Yichuanxue*, p. 223.
74 Mu Guangzong, 'Lun Zhongguo renkou de suzhi kongzhi: Guanyu Zhonghua minzu weilai de shehuixue sikao' (The control of the quality of China's population: Sociological considerations about the future of the Chinese nation), *Renkouxue*, 1991, no. 4, p. 75.

the birth of 'zero worth' beings, euthanasia should ensure
their controlled death. Cong Li, on the other hand, proposes
to screen and select (*shaixuan*) new-born babies in order to
'select the superior and discard the inferior' (*xuanyou qulie*);
this is because eugenic policies are inadequate to prevent
defective births. One of the few to consider the need for
approval from both parents, the author also wishes to confine
euthanasia strictly to grave hereditary diseases. However, as
medical knowledge concerning genetic diseases expands, it is
predicted that the number of cases to be eliminated by
euthanasia will increase, leading to an ever more eugenic
society.[75] More recently, an article written by Zhou Xianzhi,
an associate professor at the Hunan Institute for Finance and
Economics, and Li Xiaowei, a doctor attached to the
Institute's Department of Obstetrics, has also advocated
'superior death' (*yousi*) for defective children, including those
judged to be mentally retarded, as the necessary component
of a programme to ensure 'superior births' (*yousheng*).[76]

The costs of maintaining congenitally handicapped people
is often invoked to justify eugenic legislation. Chen Muhua,
vice-president of the Standing Committee of the National
People's Congress and President of the Women's Federation,
declared: 'Eugenics not only affects the success of the state
and the prosperity of the race, but also the well-being of the
people and social stability.'[77] The Eugenics Symposium over
which she presided in Beijing on 28 January 1989 judged
that more than 30 million people in the People's Republic
were genetically defective: the total cost of their maintenance was estimated at seven to eight billion yuan a year, and

75 Cong Li, 'Yousheng zhong de "shaixuan" yu daode' (Ethics and eugenic
selection), *Shandong yike daxue xuebao*, 1989, no. 2, pp. 13–14.
76 Zhou Xianzhi and Li Xiaowei, 'Shengming zhiliang dilie xinsheng'er "yousi"
tantao' (Discussion of euthanasia of infants of inferior quality), *Renkou yanjiu*,
1995, no. 3, pp. 58–61; the article was edited by Mu Guangzong.
77 *Dagongbao*, 'Zhiming renshi zuotan zhichu: tuixing yousheng ke bu rong
huan' (Public figures point out that eugenics policies are of great urgency), 30
January 1991, p. 12.

the Symposium advocated eugenic education and legislation. In another example, Gao Jinsheng, based at the Suzhou Medical Institute, estimated the costs of maintaining people suffering from 'congenital idiocy' in 1985.[78] Similar to the articles and charts depicting the costs of keeping alive the impaired at the expense of the healthy in a number of European countries throughout the 1930s, meticulous calculations are made to estimate that each patient costs exactly 25 yuan and consumes about 25 jin of cereals every month. The total costs incurred by the state thus amount to approximately 3–400 million yuan and 3–400 million jin of cereals a year. A diseased element surviving thirty to fifty years costs 10–15,000 yuan.

The first national exhibition on eugenics and the scientific control of human reproduction, entitled 'Human Reproduction and Health', which opened in the Shanghai Exhibition Centre on 23 November 1993, used graphs to illustrate the 'heavy burden' represented by the country's handicapped people.[79] In these official calculations, human life is gradually reduced to financial terms, while population health is seen as a negative balance sheet to be redressed in the interests of public well-being. The lives of disabled people are described as not worth living; they are perceived as a financial burden and a drain on public resources, and a mere figure is adduced to illustrate the useless dissipation of costly medications. Perfection is thought to reside in a set of reified medical standards.

Similar views, of course, existed in many developed countries until a few decades ago. Only very recently has the notion of a unique human value been associated with disabled infants in a small number of economically advanced societies. Eugenic programmes and sterilisation laws were an

78 Gao Jinsheng, 'Yichuanbing shi yousheng de dadi' (Hereditary diseases are the great enemy of eugenic births) in *Renkouxue*, 1985, no. 4, pp. 43–4.
79 'Profile of Shanghai exhibition views "heavy burden" of China's disabled', SWB, 1 December 1993, FE/1860 G/6.

integral part of the welfare system in Denmark, Finland, Norway and Sweden up till 1960.[80] When sterilisation acts were first passed in Sweden in 1934 and 1941, Social Democrats were the most vigorous defenders of eugenic legislation; it was thought that the systematic sterilisation of the mentally retarded would yield substantial economic gains by cutting the cost of institutional care and poor relief. An efficient administration ensured that the laws were thoroughly implemented: by 1960, well over 50,000 people had been sterilised by the initiative of the Swedish government, at first on medical grounds but later for social reasons. In Finland till recently, many medical practitioners were in favour of sterilisation and few members of the public had the desire or opportunity to dispute expert opinion. In the absence of any substantial objections, almost 2,000 people were sterilised between 1935 and 1955. In marked contrast to the commonly accepted observation that eugenics declined rapidly after the Second World War, the total number of operations performed in Finland sharply increased, and by 1970 the total had reached 56,000. With the enactment of the new Sterilisation Act and Castration Act in 1950, compulsory operations became possible with the authorisation of two doctors only.

In the 1970s, parts of the liberal intelligentsia in the Soviet Union started proposing a form of 'socialist eugenics', portraying themselves as a genetically superior élite destined by DNA to rule over the products of inferior conceptions. The systematic invocation of human genetics in political theories justifying social inequality even forced a prominent geneticist to denounce the abuse of science in an official organ of the Central Committee.[81] Eugenic arguments also surface regu-

---

80 Gunnar Broberg and Nils Roll-Hansen (eds), *Eugenics and the welfare state: Sterilization policy in Denmark, Sweden, Norway, and Finland*, East Lansing: Michigan State University Press, 1996.
81 N. Dubinin, 'Nasledovanie biologicheskoe i sotsial'noe', *Kommunist*, 11 (July 1980), pp. 62–74.

larly in the United States, as in the proposal in 1991 by state representative David Duke, a former Grand Wizard in the Ku Klux Klan, for a law offering mostly African-American female welfare recipients in Louisiana cash payments for the use of a contraceptive device called Norplant: this proposal strongly echoed earlier eugenic reforms. Forced sterilisations for eugenic reasons were performed in parts of Switzerland decades after the end of the Second World War.[82] Seen in a comparative perspective, eugenics in the PRC is not a lone exception so much as an integral part of far more widespread trends which have been and continue to be prominent in the twentieth century, although the PRC is the only powerful country officially promoting such ideas at its very end.

It could be suggested that eugenic discourse only emerged from a small group of high functionaries, while relaxations and accommodations are negotiated at local level by family planning personnel and by specialists in research institutes. However, there is ample evidence that eugenic legislation is actively supported by specialists and medical authorities at local levels: as in a number of European countries up till the 1960s, a limited number of high bureaucrats are actively supported by specific research institutions and population specialists who have been promoted to positions of power and prestige by the government after 1978. Although medical experts work under government supervision, they also exert an influence on official population policy as participants in special advisory committees, the most influential of which is the Population Advisory Committee founded by the State Family Planning Commission in July 1988.

The close relationship between research institutions and government in the PRC is well known, and formal government control and informal personal networks contribute to

82 On Switzerland, see Philippe Ehrenström, 'Stérilisation opératoire et maladie mentale. Une étude de cas', *Gesnerus*, 48 (1991), pp. 503–16, and Frank Preiswerk, 'Auguste Forel (1848–1931). Un projet de régénération sociale, morale et raciale', *Annuelles. Revue d'Histoire Contemporaine*, 2 (1991), pp. 25–50.

the integration of medical research with government policies. The data collected by research institutions are distributed only in restricted arenas of information, mainly through
personal networks, institutional connections, journals for
closed circulation, or material classified as secret. Such studies are supported at the highest level of the government, in
particular by a group of top party officials centred around Li
Peng, an open and active supporter of eugenics who was also
directly involved in the events in Tiananmen Square. The
State Family Planning Commission was one of the few
organisations that came out against eugenics.[83] Its head
Wang Wei was replaced on 22 January 1988 by Peng Peiyun,
herself a conservative cadre who was appointed Secretary of
the Party after the purge of Fang Lizhi at Hefei University of
Science and Technology, and confirmed as Head by Li Peng
on 12 April 1988. Chen Muhua, chair of a Eugenics
Symposium in 1989, and Chen Minzhang, the Minister of
Public Health who proposed the eugenics law, both have
close ties to Li Peng, confirming the impression that eugenic
policies are supported by a small fraction of conservative
party officials. Qian Xinzhong, another high party official
who served as Honorary President of the Medical
Association and Honorary President of the Ultrasonic
Medicine Society among other posts, was made President of
the Eugenics Society in January 1989, and his calligraphy
regularly endorses publications which directly promote
applied eugenics.[84]

Outside the government, different medical fields, from
embryology to cytogenetics, have become responsible for
providing the government with medical knowledge on the
incidence and control of 'inferior births'. The genetics lobby,
far from resisting the use of science in the politics of quality

83 Nicholas D. Kristof, 'Parts of China forcibly sterilizing the retarded who wish
to marry', *New York Times*, 15 August 1991, p. 1.
84 For instance Yan Renying and Lin Guimei, *Shiyong yousheng shouce*
(Handbook of applied eugenics), Beijing: Renmin weisheng chubanshe, 1992.

control, has been at the forefront of a campaign for eugenic legislation since the late 1970s. The need to restore genetics as a prominent field of research after the debacle of the Great Leap Forward and the Cultural Revolution, the desire for professional status and opportunities for greater financial resources, the naive exaltation of 'science' as a unified system able to provide the ultimate truth in all domains, the domination over research of strict social hierarchies, patronage systems and master-disciple relations in which gerontocrats define the parameters of acceptable research – these are some of the reasons why geneticists have actively pushed rather than passively followed the government towards the enactment of a eugenics law. Among other factors for the active involvement of geneticists in eugenics are the resistance to new research hypotheses and the resilience of older theoretical frames of reference, which are seen as of better pedigree and thus of higher value. Furthermore, the written word is held in great respect, including outdated if not antiquated publications from the 1960s which are still referred to. Even eugenic writings from the 1930s have been rehabilitated: ostracised for decades as a 'rightist' element, Pan Guangdan is not only hailed as China's father of eugenics in popular literature, but his works from the republican period are uncritically recommended for their 'scientific value' even in *Hereditas*, the leading journal of the genetics' community.[85]

As concern over population quality has gradually spread since the late 1970s, medical science has been able to attract significant amounts of money to be spent on research facilities and sophisticated medical equipment. Under the auspices of the Chinese Academy of Science, a Centre for

85 Liu Jinxiang, 'Ping Pan Guangdan de *Yousheng gailun*' (A review of Pan Guangdan's *Introduction to eugenics*), *Yichuan*, 1982, no. 3, pp. 39–40; in demography, see Hu Jize, 'Yao dong yidian youshengxue (jieshao Pan Guangdan de *Yousheng yuanli*)' (We should understand some eugenics: Introducing Pan Guangdan's *Eugenic principles*), *Renkouxue*, 1986, no. 3, pp. 74–6.

Developmental Biology was established at the end of the 1970s by Professor Niu Manjiang for the advancement of positive eugenics. The Population Research Institute of Anhui University was officially recognised in 1987 as a centre for the study of eugenics, and the People's University, Nanjing University and Zhejiang Medical University have been engaged in the study of 'population quality' since the end of the 1980s. National Medical Genetics Centres were also established in Beijing, Shanghai and Hunan. A fourth centre was opened in January 1989 in Inner Mongolia with the specific aim of ameliorating the 'quality' of the minority populations.[86] Moreover, a China Birth Defect Monitoring Centre in Chengdu was made responsible for directing eugenics at a national level. Pilot projects responsible for closely monitoring birth defects in thirty counties have been set up by the State Family Planning Commission, and the Ministry of Health organised the systematic screening for birth defects of over 1,240,000 children in 945 different hospitals between October 1986 and September 1987, providing medical and government circles with practical experience for a more widespread implementation of eugenic programmes. For the sake of achieving a healthier nation and a eugenic future, learned journals routinely publish surveys of scanning techniques, diagnoses of birth defects and ways to abort malformed foetuses.[87] In teratological

86 *Dagongbao*, 'Yixue yichuan yanjiu zhongxin. Zai Nei Meng zizhiqu chengli' (Medical genetics research centre established in the Inner Mongolia Autonomous Region), 29 January 1989, p. 6.

87 Some of the most prestigious journals are the *Journal of Medical Ultrasonics* (*Zhongguo chaosheng yixue zazhi*), *Hereditas* (*Yichuan*) and the *Chinese Journal of Family Planning* (*Zhongguo jihua shengyu zazhi*). While some articles are specifically concerned with severe defects, others concentrate on mild defects; a typical example is Cao Shaoman, 'Chaosheng xianxiang zhenduan tai'er chunlie jixing' (Ultrasonic diagnosis of the hare-lip defect in the foetus), *Zhongguo chaosheng yixue zazhi*, 1995, no. 10, pp. 770–2, in which the author reports to have scanned 3,177 cases during the 22nd week, having detected the three offending cases 'without fail'.

research, an important landmark was the publication in 1993 of the first systematic medical report on embryological development and the prevention of birth defects, involving more than 300 specialists from seventy work units.[88] As noted throughout this chapter, the child care orientation of screening technologies may not be substantially different from similar endeavours in developed countries. What differs is the overall eugenic framework within which these technologies are used, and their inadequate accountability: they may be biased towards the eugenics lobby regardless of the wishes of the women concerned.

Since the end of the Cultural Revolution, while financial resources dedicated to genetic research in the coastal cities have increased, health care in the poorer regions of the hinterland has gradually deteriorated. Marked by a shift from preventive to curative health care on the one hand and by a change of emphasis from the countryside to the cities, the inequalities between rich city people and poor country dwellers has increased since 1978.[89] With the economic reforms initiated by Deng Xiaoping, the government has significantly reduced its support for health services, forcing hospitals to focus on profit-making services for wealthy inpatients at the expense of health care for the underprivileged and vulnerable outpatients. As access to basic health care becomes increasingly inequitable, the burden of infant and maternal health care has shifted away from the government towards families. The cheap but relatively efficient health care system set up in the countryside after 1949 has all but collapsed, and many small villages are left to their own devices to survive. Many poor peasants cannot pay even for

88 Gu Huayun (ed.), *Zhongguoren peitai fayu shixu he jitai yufang* (The development of the embryo in Chinese people and the prevention of malformations), Shanghai: Yike daxue chubanshe, 1993.
89 On this topic see Veronica Pearson, 'Health and responsibility: But whose?' in Linda Wong and Steward MacPherson (eds), *Social change and social policy in China*, Aldershot: Avebury, 1995, pp. 88–112.

basic treatment, let alone for the expensive operations that are necessary when medical complications occur with babies. Rather than recognising that the economic reforms have created significant health problems in the countryside, the campaigns in reproductive health conveniently blame dispossessed and marginalised people for their own poor health, emphasising their 'defective genes', 'inborn deficiencies' as well as 'feudal customs' – as this chapter has sought to demonstrate. Eugenic discourse has created a large consensus among social groups with a voice, from local cadres, the urban middle classes and medical groups to academic circles. Marginalised and impoverished people, from small farmer villages in Gansu province to minority people in Tibet, have had little if any opportunity to express their dissent.

However, since the late 1980s disagreement with eugenic ideas and practices has been disregarded even in the coastal cities. In a number of surveys on attitudes towards severely disabled babies carried out by Chinese researchers interested in medical ethics in the second half of the 1980s, it appeared that up to 25% of those questioned considered life to be sacred in all circumstances. In one survey, 12% believed that even babies with exceptionally severe handicaps destined to an early death should still be given medical treatment, while 23% were in favour of extensive assistance for children born without limbs. On the other hand, up to 15% supported the termination of cases with mild handicaps which could be medically corrected; a cleft palate was given as an example of this level of disability.[90] Asked whether babies with severe handicaps should be allowed to die by withdrawing medical assistance, nearly a quarter of interviewees in Beijing in 1990, drawn from a variety of social backgrounds, considered life to be sacred and equated lack of medical assistance

---

90 Pan Ronghua and Zhou Xiaojun, '448 ren dui quexian xinsheng'er de chuli diaocha baogao' (Report on an investigation of 448 persons' attitudes towards the treatment of disabled neonates), *Yixue yu zhexue*, 1988, no. 3, pp. 28–30.

with murder.[91] These opinion polls, however problematic epistemologically and methodologically, indicate that a significant percentage of people find the 'disposal' of infants with disabilities highly objectionable. While these surveys generally play down these contradictory results by representing eugenics as a practice supported by 'the great majority' of the population, they nonetheless reveal that attitudes towards disability are as complex in China as elsewhere, despite the very limited information and social support publicly available to those who depart from official views.

The termination by euthanasia of babies deemed unfit was also criticised in 1985 in an article of *Medicine and Philosophy*, a journal which has pioneered work in medical ethics. Signed by Yang Nairong, it disagreed with the legal, ethical and medical considerations invoked to justify consensual infanticide.[92] The article, however, was quickly rebutted in the same journal by a doctor from Dalian Hospital, who hailed the advantages of mercy-killing in the implementation of a thorough eugenics programme, on the grounds that the control and disposal of 'unfit genes' would be conducive to a fitter future.[93] Qiu Renzong, Professor at the Philosophy Institute of the Chinese Academy of Social Sciences, has been an even more significant voice raised in defence of ethical considerations in eugenic discourse. He has insisted on the right of individuals and their families to refuse sterilisation or termination of pregnancy; explicitly extended these

91 Liu Shijing *et al.*, 'Beijing shi 360 ming butong renqun dui you quexian xinsheng'er chuli yijian de diaocha yu fenxi' (Investigation and analysis of the attitudes towards the treatment of disabled neonates of 360 people of different social backgrounds in Beijing municipality), *Zhongguo yixue lunlixue*, 1990, no. 10, pp. 29–30.

92 Yang Nairong, 'Bu ying sheqi yanzhong xiantian quexian binghuan er' (Against the abandonment of severely congenitally handicapped neonates), *Yixue yu zhexue*, 1985, no. 6, p. 49.

93 Wang Xiangchu, 'Ye lun dui yanzhong xiantian quexian binghuan er de sheqi' (Again about the abandonment of severely congenitally handicapped neonates), *Yixue yu zhexue*, 1985, no. 11, pp. 53–5.

rights to those defined as 'mentally retarded'; questioned the criteria whereby entire categories of people are dismissed as 'unfit' or 'deficient'; and denounced the stereotypical language used by medical experts when writing of people with mental or physical disabilities.[94] Despite these isolated voices, it is clear that eugenics generally reflects the desire of a majority of doctors and cadres to be freed from a 'burden'. To concentrate on a small number of dissenting individuals and dwell on the occasional 'contestation' in order to highlight a presumed 'diversity' of social positions in this debate could convey a seriously distorted image. The influence on policy-making of critically inclined individuals is limited, and such people do not represent a majority among the experts in positions of power who contribute to the dominant eugenic discourse. Under a one-party regime which does not encourage the expression of marginalised voices, ideas of 'social contestation' or even 'informed choice' do not have much tangible reality.

As the result of such consensus, local regulations have been passed virtually unopposed in a number of provinces and cities since the late 1980s. Although calls for a marital ban on certain categories of people appeared in the *People's Daily* as early as 1980 ('imbeciles, lunatics, haemophiliacs and those who are colour-blind or carry hereditary disease'),[95] the first eugenic laws were only passed at the provincial level at the end of the decade. The *People's Daily* announced on 25 November 1988 that the Standing Committee of the National People's Congress of Gansu Province had passed the country's first law prohibiting mentally retarded people from having children.[96] The article reported that Gansu

94 See, for instance, Qiu Renzong, 'Dui zhili yanzhong dixiazhe shixing jueyu de lunlixue wenti' (Some ethical questions about the sterilisation of severely retarded people), *Zhongguo yixue lunlixue*, 1992, no. 1, pp. 10–15.

95 Zhong Hulan, *Renmin ribao*, 21 May 1980.

96 'Gansu tongguo difang fagui jinzhi chidai sharen shengyu' (Gansu province promulgates a law prohibiting mentally retarded people to bear children), *Renmin ribao*, 25 November 1988.

province counted more than 270,000 'feeble-minded' people, breeding approximately 2,000 retarded children each year. According to the law, those mentally retarded people whose condition was either inherited or a consequence of marriage between close relatives were not allowed to have children; no mentally retarded people were allowed to get married unless they had undergone sterilisation surgery; those who had married before the promulgation of the law were also to undergo sterilisation surgery; and pregnant women suffering from mental retardation were required to have their pregnancies terminated. Individuals who violated the law by allowing mentally retarded people to have children would be punished by both administrative and economic means.[97] A similar law was enacted by Liaoning province in February 1990, while Zhejiang province passed a law on the preservation of 'eugenic health' in June 1992 to combat the increasing incidence of 'cretins', who were estimated to number more than 300,000.[98] The Henan eugenics law of 1992 requires that if one partner in a married couple suffers from a 'chronic mental disorder' such as schizophrenia or manic depression, that partner shall be sterilised. The implementation of such sterilisation laws at the provincial level is advanced by a system of incentives and disincentives. Incentives often consist of additional paid maternity leave. People who refuse to be sterilised or anyone who impedes the sterilisation of another may be subject to penalties. For example, Henan's eugenics law requires prompt reporting of those diagnosed as 'needing to be sterilised' who refuse to accept the operation. Differential fines for non-compliance

97 A closer look at the law can be found in Harro von Senger, 'Erbgesundheitslehre in der Volksrepublik China' in Jarmila Bedbaríková and Frank C. Chapmann (eds), *Festschrift für Jan Stepán*, Zürich: Schulthess Polygraphischer Verlag, 1994, pp. 219–32.
98 'Zhejiang sheng yousheng baojian tiaoli' (Zhejiang province's regulations in eugenics and the protection of health), *Renkou yu yousheng*, 1992, no. 3, p. 5.

with 'eugenic measures' are imposed for rural and urban residents.[99]

Under pressure from a variety of lobbies, mainly family planning experts and geneticists, the provincial laws finally culminated in the People's Republic of China passing eugenic legislation at the national level at the beginning of 1995. As this law has been commented upon in great detail by a number of observers,[100] it will be sufficient to summarise its main aspects briefly, while emphasising yet again that the different meanings of eugenics in China can only be understood in the broader social, cultural and political context which this book has attempted to analyse. The law, as is well known, aims to prevent 'inferior births' from becoming a burden on the state and society. Renamed 'Maternal and Infant Health Law' after protests against a preliminary draft entitled 'Eugenics Law', it supports the systematic 'implementation of premarital medical check-ups' in order to detect whether one partner in a couple suffers from a 'serious hereditary', venereal or reproductive disorder, a 'relevant mental disorder' or a 'legal contagious disease': it asserts that those 'deemed unsuitable for reproduction' should be urged to undergo sterilisation or abortion, or to remain celibate, in order to prevent 'inferior births'.[101] During pregnancy, prenatal testing will be compulsory and can be

---

99 See the Henan Eugenics Health Protection Regulations of August 1992, translated in *Joint Publications Research Service*, 22 December 1992, p. 47.

100 Among others, see Elisabeth J. Croll, 'A commentary on the new draft law on eugenics and health protection', *China Information*, 8, no. 3 (winter 1993–4), pp. 32–7; of special interest is Dagmar Borchard, 'Aus einem Melonenkern entsteht eine Melone. Gesetzliche Rahmenbedingungen der Eugenik', *Das Neue China*, 1994, no. 4, pp. 25–7; on the recent legislation on marriage registration, which is an important means of implementing eugenic measures, see Dagmar Borchard, 'VR China. Neue Vorschriften zur Kontrolle der Eheregistrierung', *Das Standesamt*, 49, no. 2 (Sept. 1996), pp. 275–80.

101 'Zhonghua renmin gongheguo muying baojian fa' (The People's Republic of China's maternal and infant health law), *Zhonghua renmin gongheguo quanguo renmin daibiao dahui changwu weiyuanhui gongbao*, 1994, no. 7, pp. 3–8.

followed by termination if the foetus is found to have a serious disorder.

SOCIAL AND ETHICAL IMPLICATIONS
OF POPULATION POLICIES

The most striking aspect of eugenic legislation is no doubt its compulsory character: genetic considerations are invoked to curb an individual's reproductive freedom for the sake of public health. Contrary to the provincial sterilisation laws, the 1995 law explicitly points to voluntary sterilisation: the question is what importance can possibly be given to 'individual choice' in a one-party state that has never hesitated to imprison citizens who disagree with official policy, or indeed to use military force to suppress student dissent, as happened in Tiananmen Square in June 1989. One may wonder how much weight is likely to be given to personal wishes when one is talking of people defined as 'mentally ill' and others deemed by medical authorities and local cadres to be 'unfit', and how this wish can be respected without the legal framework necessary to safeguard it. It is easy to slip from voluntary to compulsory sterilisation, and one fundamental difference between genetic counselling and eugenics is precisely that the former informs families of potential risks whereas the latter instructs them whether or not they may have children. The coercive implementation of birth control programmes so far indicates that eugenic legislation will be carried out with little regard for individual choice.

Another troublesome aspect of eugenic legislation is that the right to reproduce and even the right to exist are determined by ill-defined and partial ideas about 'genetic fitness'. Eugenic discourse suffers from a lack of a clear definition of what constitutes or should be considered a 'severe' handicap. Down's syndrome and hydrocephalus are often cited as examples of 'severe inherited diseases', but so are haemophilia, mucopolysaccharidosis and even diabetes: it has been suggested that foetuses which are found by a DNA test after the first four months of pregnancy to be affected by any of these disorders should be 'instantly aborted'.[102] No definition is provided for the terms 'mental retardation' and 'mental illness', which are often used in official statements and eugenic legislation. There is a wide range of mental disabilities, many of them only partly understood, and few forms of mental illness can be demonstrated as clearly having a genetic cause, yet both political and medical authorities unhesitatingly prescribe sterilisation for those judged to be 'retarded'. Although information about the enforcement of the eugenics laws is not forthcoming from tight-lipped local and national officials, most decisions on who is and is not unfit to reproduce are apparently left to local doctors, many of whom have no more than a high-school education.[103] The eugenics law effectively gives considerable power over people's reproductive rights to unit cadres and local doctors, and this inevitably increases corruption and bureaucratic incompetence as people try to obtain marriage licences.[104]

Although it is clear that in the poorer regions of China many people suffer from a variety of severe mental problems, 'mental retardation' itself is a social definition that reflects socially agreed norms and expectations rather than an objective set of medical criteria. The treatment of those socially defined as mentally retarded is, more often than not, defined by the negative meaning of that term rather than by the needs and situations of particular individuals. 'Retardants' are seen in the PRC as a menace to the health of society and a burden on its charity. Based on the notion that intellectual capacity is unalterable, few attempts are made to approach

---

102 Zhao Gongmin, *Yichuanxue yu shehui* (Genetics and society), Shenyang: Liaoning renmin chubanshe, 1986, p. 214.
103 Nicolas D. Kristof, 'Parts of China forcibly sterilizing the retarded who wish to marry', *New York Times*, 15 August 1991, p. 1.
104 Lincoln Kaye, 'Quality control: Eugenics bill defended against Western critics', *Far Eastern Economic Review*, 13 January 1994, p. 22.

those defined as retarded as developing individuals to be helped and rehabilitated. The popular literature on family health tends to expatiate on medical norms which remain elusive to most poor people outside the big cities, rather than providing such people with useful information on how they could alleviate congenital disabilities. It offers precious little help to the parents of mentally disabled children.[105] In that sense the widespread use of value terms and stereotypic language in both medical and popular discourse says more about social prejudices than about particular handicaps. In China as elsewhere, there is a wide range of mental disability which resists the use of generic terms, and those afflicted by these disabilities often display emotions and temperaments similar to those of the rest of the population.

Such loose definitions of 'mental retardation' lead to the sterilisation of thousands of individuals. Although precise figures may never be obtainable, an article published in May 1993 in the People's Daily claimed that 2,000 people in Gansu had been sterilised since the implementation of the 1988 law.[106] The real figure is undoubtedly much higher, and it remains to be established how many women have been coerced into undergoing sterilisation or forced abortion in China following similar provincial laws. Some provinces, of course, do not have such laws and may even disregard the 1995 national law. With political power shifting from the centre to the provinces, some regions may implement existing laws quite strictly while others completely ignore them. Furthermore, some local cadres may be reluctant to impose reproductive restrictions on parents with a handicapped child: many proponents of eugenic legislation complain

105 One of the few articles on rehabilation is Qiu Jinghua, 'Ruozhi ertong de kangfu xunlian' (Rehabilitation exercices for mildly retarded children), Jiankang shijie, 1996, no. 6, pp. 16–17.
106 Dagmar Borchard, 'Aus einem Melonenkern entsteht eine Melone: Gesetzliche Rahmenbedingungen der Eugenik', Das Neue China, 1994, no. 4, pp. 25–27.

about the ignorance of some local workers, who allow couples who give birth to a baby with a birth defect to have another child. Unfortunately, in the absence of any detailed studies by social anthropologists and population experts, concrete information on the implementation of eugenic laws is missing.

The crucial point, however, is that the government only in the early 1990s started to recognise that a lack of iodine, rather than 'defective' genes, is at the root of many problems of mental health in the countryside. This particular deficiency, in China as in other developing countries, causes chronic mental and physical fatigue as well as varying degrees of mental impairment. While most governments have long taken remedial steps by adding trace amounts of iodine to table salt, the party leadership has belatedly yielded to continuous pressure from international agencies and recognised the problem. However, evidence indicates that the sale of iodised salt from some government distribution centres has fallen as non-iodised salt remains a cheaper option in poor regions of the country.[107]

Even when lack of iodine has been identified as a major factor in the prevalence of mental retardation, eugenic measures continue to be justified on the grounds of lack of parental responsibility towards their offspring of cretins. The confusion between hereditary, congenital and acquired diseases also works in favour of eugenic measures, as the author of one of the earliest articles on iodine deficiency concluded: 'Some scholars wonder why reproduction should be restricted if cretinism is not hereditary. This writer believes that eugenics should be implemented even where non-hereditary diseases are concerned. The scope of modern eugenics has already gone beyond the simple consideration of the biological quality of offspring from the point of view of genetics: one has to guarantee the health of future generations through

107 Patrick E. Tyler, 'Lacking iodine in their diets, millions in China are retarded', *New York Times*, 4 June 1996, p. A1.

the prevention of all sorts of non-hereditary congenital diseases [*fei yichuan de xiantian jibing*].'[108] Lack of folic acid, another scourge which is not adequately addressed in China, is also responsible for major health problems when it occurs in the first month of foetal life, since it can lead to severe deformities of the spinal cord. While an urgent programme was developed in the early 1990s thanks to foreign assistance, the absence of systematic provision of iodine and folic acid has left the population at risk. On the other hand, expensive and sophisticated medical equipment is regularly purchased by the hospitals in the coastal cities to screen pregnant mothers for this or that relatively rare 'genetic disease': thus lack of financial resources hardly adequately explains the authorities' reluctance to advocate and educate the worst affected areas vigorously in the need for these crucial nutrients.

The example of mental retardation illustrates the human cost of the confusions that are frequently and deliberately made in China between the dietary, environmental and genetic factors of population health. Although, to take another example, 'deafness' is portrayed as a 'grave hereditary defect', it is well-known that this condition can arise from a multiplicity of factors, only half of which are hereditary. Moreover, as more than thirty distinct genes are involved in cases of inborn deafness, many parents with normal hearing produce a deaf child while deaf people from different families may have a child with normal hearing.[109] What appears a simple matter is often far more complex, ambiguous and uncertain than eugenic discourse would have it. Even when a disease may have a genetic element, it is only rarely acknowledged that 'fitness' and 'defectiveness' are only relative concepts, and not intrinsic genetic properties.

---

108 Zhang Chunqing and Liu Guirong, 'Kedingbing huanzhe de hunyu yu yousheng lifa' (Cretinism and marriage in the light of eugenic legislation), *Yixue yu zhexue*, 1991, no. 8, pp. 44–5.
109 Steve Jones, *In the blood: God, genes and destiny*, London: HarperCollins, 1996, p. 33.

In other words, the implementation of eugenic legislation does not only undermine the rights of the person vis-à-vis the state, but it is based on controversial if not antiquated theories: even in those rare cases of a demonstrable one-to-one correspondence between a gene and a defect, sterilisation will not significantly reduce the incidence of mental illness in the population. If a genetic trait is recessive or polygenic, sterilisation is a utopian measure, in particular since a person with mental disability by reason of heredity is more often than not the offspring of normal parents. Even to rid people in Britain of the recessive form of PKU, as Lionel Penrose calculated more than half a century ago, 1 per cent of the British population would have to be sterilised.[110]

Moreover, discredited eugenic theories assume that population groups are static and that genetic traits all originate in a particular line of descent. Already in the 1930s, both J.B.S. Haldane and Penrose surmised that some disorders arise not principally from hereditary transmission, but from random mutations. The absence of clear definitions of health and ill-health in China's eugenic legislation logically entails that the reproduction of every single individual should be controlled, since every human being is the bearer of some sort of 'defective' gene. This suggests that the reasons for promoting such legislation may have more to do with politics than with medicine, because of the considerable power it gives to local cadres and medical experts. This suspicion is strengthened by the insertion of a clause in the 1995 law which states that it is sufficient for a doctor merely to 'suspect' a pregnant women of foetal abnormality to recommend diagnostic tests and possibly termination of the pregnancy. Moreover, in many ways, the law may do no more than condone an established practice, since doctors are likely to eliminate children at birth who have visible defects without telling the parents, as was

110 D.J. Kevles, *In the name of eugenics: Genetics and the use of human heredity*, New York: Alfred Knopf, 1985, p. 288.

common in developed countries until the 1960s.[111] In the bigger hospitals, ethical committees have been set up to adjudicate over difficult ethical issues, although they are run by the hospital administration which is dominated by party members inclined to apply the official population policies. The families concerned have little say in vital decisions taken by doctors and cadres; furthermore, eugenic measures are constantly justified by invoking the welfare of future generations. Abstractions like the 'race', 'future generations' and the 'gene pool' are elevated above the rights and needs of individuals and their families, just as claims about 'the state', 'the revolution' or 'the party' have been used in the past in ideological movements.

Furthermore, eugenic discourse colludes with patrilineal culture, in particular folk models of inheritance which see disorders as running in family lines. The lack of any serious effort to establish guidelines on what constitutes a 'birth defect' is compounded by gender prejudice, in particular the cultural preference for a son: a female embryo may be considered a defect in itself. As screening techniques, in particular the use of ultrasound detectors, are routinely used in many parts of the coastal region, the sex ratio in favour of boys has been skewed even further. Although the government has issued a ban on tests to determine the sex of an embryo, doctors readily accept gifts to detect and abort female foetuses: in two cities in Shandong province, Chinese researchers themselves have reported a 10 − 1 male-female ratio for the second child.[112] The number of abandoned children since the 1970s with minor defects such as a harelip or a cleft palate − both of which only require a minor surgical operation to be corrected − has been significant over the

111 See Martin S. Pernick, *The black stork: Eugenics and the death of 'defective' babies in American medicine and motion pictures since 1915*, Oxford University Press, 1996.
112 Liu Qi, 'Tai'er xingbie jianding jishu yingyong de lunli daode wenti' (Ethical questions on the use of tests for prenatal sex determination), *Zhongguo yixue lunlixue*, 1995, no. 2, pp. 46–7.

past two decades, further suggesting that social prejudice against babies with birth defects is important.[113] Although euthanasia has not yet been officially approved as a medical practice, there is mounting evidence that abandoned children with real or presumed disabilities are deliberately selected for 'summary resolution' by way of death by starvation. Some deaths from malnutrition of otherwise healthy children in orphanages are retrospectively recorded as 'cerebral palsy' or 'congenital maldevelopment of the brain'.[114] Although far more evidence would be necessary to evaluate how common this is, it nonetheless indicates how eugenic legislation could provide a legal framework for controversial social practices.

Historically, scientific advances in genetic research have brought mankind not only greater knowledge of human reproduction, but also increased social prejudice against racial, sexual, religious or political minorities, leading to sterilisation programmes against devalued individuals. While the crude eugenic approaches described in this chapter may be unique to the PRC, the legacy of eugenics is still highly visible also in developed countries, mainly in contemporary debates about new medical techniques for isolating and manipulating genes. Gene therapy, embryo selection and prenatal screening are important tools which are open to race and class bias, threatening a commitment to social equality and reproductive rights. Information about human genetics can be used to stigmatise not only people alleged to suffer from genetic diseases, but almost anybody whose exis-

113 Zhang Juan and Qin Chao, '296 li shangcan qi'er de shengming lunlixue fenxi' (Bioethical analysis on 296 cases of abandoned children with disabilities), *Yixue yu zhexue*, 1989, no. 8, pp. 30–2; see also Kay Johnson, 'Chinese orphanages: Saving China's abandoned girls', *Australian Journal of Chinese Studies*, no. 30 (July 1993), pp. 61–87.
114 Human Rights Watch, *Death by default: A policy of fatal neglect in China's state orphanages*, Human Rights Watch Report, January 1996.

tence is deemed to be economically costly or socially undesirable.

During the heyday of eugenics, assumptions about 'race', sex and class pervaded genetic research: with the revolution in human genetics in our own time, social and political factors continue to exert formidable influence on scientific research, although eugenic laws are unlikely to reappear in countries which protect reproductive freedoms and civil rights. However, it is true that even in democratic countries, marginalised people may be treated in a discriminatory way, as social prejudice and economic interest are liable to affect the exact nature of the genetic information made available to families, employers, hospitals, insurance companies or welfare systems. Exploring the history of eugenics thus illuminates how sterilisation laws in the PRC are an integral part of more global trends which have deeply marked and continue to affect the twentieth century. Whether or not it is likely to help us undermine the credibility of eugenics in that country is open to debate.

5

CONCLUSION

The advantage of an historical methodology which distinguishes between credibility and validity, and is interested more in an inductive investigation of the specific causes of a statement's general acceptance than in its epistemological status as true or false, resides in its ability to show the radically contingent and partial nature of medical knowledge.[1] This is not to say that all knowledge is equally true or equally false, for this would mean abandoning the possibility of challenging and criticising medical knowledge on its own terms; it is merely to say that different scientific approaches, necessarily grounded in cultural, social and political contingencies, lead to the discovery of very different types of evidence. Gendered discourse which represented women as the passive counterparts of men privileged sperm as the only active agent in medical descriptions of the fertilisation process, positively and effectively leading to the discovery of the molecular mechanisms of sperm activity. Each of these 'facts' in turn consolidated a gendered version of social reality which ignored the active mechanisms by which the egg produced the proteins or molecules responsible for enabling and preventing adhesion and penetration.[2] It may well be true that scientific givens indicate that men and women are anatomically and physiologically different, but such statements cannot be seen as existing independently from a particular social context which has created the conditions for their appearance and the possibility for their expression; nor can they

3 See Barry Baines and David Bloor, 'Relativism, rationalism and the sociology of knowledge', in Martin Hollis and Steven Lukes (eds), *Rationality and relativism*, Oxford: Blackwell, 1982, pp. 21–47.
4 Evelyn Fox Keller, *Refiguring life: Metaphors of twentieth-century biology*, New York: Columbia University Press, 1995, pp. xii–xiii.

provide a legitimate basis for unequal treatment or exclusionary practices. Science cannot be expected simply to produce value-free and factual knowledge, and it cannot be used as a valid basis for prescriptive claims about social order.

As the history of eugenics shows, reliance on scientific knowledge and expert opinion without due respect for reproductive rights leads to damaging social policies. Scientific knowledge cannot be relied on to solve social problems, especially outside of a democratic political system. The conclusion to the last chapter indicates that the contingent determinants of all medical knowledge lie not so much in the inherent 'truth' of a set of given 'facts', but rather in the social and political context which endows such facts with meaning and constructs what is seen as constituting knowledge in the first place. The cultural values, social goals and political interests of such knowledge are thus to be highlighted, rather than the rationality or irrationality of particular beliefs. A variety of eugenic practices have been legitimised on the basis of medical knowledge in post-Mao China. Medical knowledge, represented as a unified and homogeneous system of absolute truth rather than a set of relative, limited and sometimes contradictory statements, is supported by established institutions and cultural authorities in the PRC who have a vested interest in the control of human reproduction.

However, the precise articulations of medical discourse in a one-party state are themselves based on more stable cultural values that transcend short-term social and political conjunctures. Below the surface of political events, beyond the cycles of social and economic change, new ideas are often produced out of old ideas. The interconnectedness of body and mind, the interdependence of self and other, the complementarity of the person with the environment – these are cultural values which have not so much been displaced as reinforced by the selective appropriation of medical knowledge from modernising countries. A discourse of descent, which links the person to his ancestors in terms of a lineage, as well as gendered ideas which propose essential differences between men and women, have also been rearticulated and enriched by new medical vocabularies.

Cultural appropriation, intentionally or unintentionally, also entails cultural transformation. Medical discourse has increasingly represented the physical body as a relatively autonomous entity with its own boundaries, focused on its inner mechanisms at the expense of cosmological forces, and stressed an ontological conception of disease in which pathological agents responsible for ill-health can be controlled. In this overdetermined universe, more open explanations, which might point to the unpredictability of birth defects and the randomness of genetic mutations, are abandoned in favour of causal interpretations which often assign a clear responsibility to individuals. Individual agency has been overemphasised by medical determinism. Moreover, from the late nineteenth century onwards, the individual has been subordinated to the nation in the name of the collective health of future generations. Science has been used by modernising intellectuals to portray each person as an organic unit belonging to a larger collectivity, called 'race', 'nation', 'state' or even 'gene pool'.

Although the individual has been attributed duties and responsibilities rather than rights and choices, the greater emphasis on personal particularities – for instance in terms of genetic status or DNA profile – can only strengthen a sense of individuality which different political regimes have suppressed. As has happened in other cases, most notably in post-war Germany and more recently in Taiwan, an organic vision of the body politic in which the duties of people are stressed at the expense of their rights can alternate with, and even lead to, new democratising trends, in which the equivalence and rights of all individuals are theoretically recognised. For such a political transformation to succeed on the mainland, however, would require a commitment to democratic goals which may well be incompatible with the narrower concerns of the intellectual and political élites.

BIBLIOGRAPHY

PRIMARY SOURCES

Late Imperial China

Cai Lin 蔡璘, *Taichan zhibao* 胎產至寶 (Essentials of childbirth), orig. 1789, 1961 edn.

Cao Tingdong 曹庭棟, *Laolao hengyan* 老老恆言 (Abiding words on the treatment of elderly people), orig. 1784, 1878 edn.

Cao Wuji 曹無極, *Wanyu xianshu* 萬育仙書 (Eternal book on childbirth), orig. 1565, Beijing: Zhongyi guji chubanshe, 1987.

Chen Fuzheng 陳復正, *Youyou jicheng* 幼幼集成 (Compendium for infant health care), orig. 1750, Shanghai: Shanghai keji chubanshe, 1962.

Chen Hu'an 陳笏庵, *Taichan jinzhen* 胎產金針 (Essentials of childbirth), orig. 1795, 1862 edn, also called *Taichan mishu* (Book of secrets on childbirth).

Chen Shiduo 陳士鐸, *Bianzhenglu* 辯症录 (Writings on medicine), orig. 1687, Beijing: Renmin weisheng chubanshe, 1965.

——, *Shishi milu* 石室秘錄 (Secret records of the Stone Chamber), orig. 1687, 1805 edn.

——, *Taichan mishu* 胎產秘書 (Book of secrets on childbirth), orig. 1687, Beijing: Renmin weisheng chubanshe, 1965.

Chen Xiuyuan 陳修園, *Nüke yaozhi* 女科要旨 (Essentials of medicine for women), orig. 1803, repr. in *Chen Xiuyuan yishu qishier zhong* 陳修園遺書七十二種 (Seventy-two medical books from Chen Xiuyuan), Shanghai: Dadong shuju, 1936.

Chen Ziming 陳自明, *Furen daquan liangfang* 婦人大全良方 (Compendium of useful prescriptions for women), orig. 1239, Beijing: Renmin chubanshe, 1985.

Dashengbian 達生編 (Book on successful childbirth), orig. 1715, Shanghai: Foxue shuju, 1934.

Fuke mishu 婦科秘書 (Book of secrets on medicine for women) in Zhu Jianping *et al.* (eds) 竹劍平, *Fuke mishu bazhong* 婦科秘書八種 (Eight secret books on medicine for women), Beijing: Zhongyi guji chubanshe, 1986.

Fuke wenda 婦科問答 (Questions and answers on medicine for women) in Zhu Jianping *et al.* (eds) 竹劍平, *Fuke mishu bazhong* 婦科秘書八種 (Eight secret books on medicine for women), Beijing: Zhongyi guji chubanshe, 1986.

Fu Shan 傅山, *Fu Qingzhu nanke* 傅青主男科 (Fu Shan's medicine for men), Shanxi kexue jishu chubanshe, 1987.

187

Huang Tizhai 黃惕齋, *Taichan jiyao* 胎產輯要 (Essentials of childbirth), orig. 1756, 1839 edn.

Jiachuan nüke jingyan zhaiqi 家傳女科經驗摘奇 (Strange passages from passed-on experiences in medicine for women) in Zhu Jianping *et al.* (eds) 竹劍平, *Fuke mishu bazhong* 婦科秘書八種 (Eight secret books on medicine for women), Beijing: Zhongyi guji chubanshe, 1986.

Ke Jia 柯㛤, *Baochan jiyao* 保產機要 (Essentials of childbirth) in *Hecuan dashengpian baochan jiyao* (Two medical works on successful childbirth), orig. 1779 edn.

Li Changke 李長科, *Taichan husheng pian* 胎產護生篇 (On childbirth and the protection of life), orig. 1798, 1862 edn.

Li Shizhen 李時珍, *Bencao gangmu* 本草綱目 (Compendium of materia medica), orig. 1578, Beijing: Renmin weisheng chubanshe, 1981.

Ling De 凌德, *Nüke zhezhong cuanyao* 女科摺衷纂要 (Essentials of medicine for women), orig. 1892, repr. in *Lidai zhongyi zhenben jicheng* 歷代中醫真本集成 (Collection of rare books on Chinese medicine), Shanghai: Sanlian shudian, 1990.

Ni Zhiwei 倪技維, *Chanbao* 產寶 (Treasure of childbirth), orig. 1728, Shanghai: Shijie shuju, 1936.

Shan Nanshan 單南山, *Taichan zhinan* 胎產指南 (Guide to childbirth), orig. 1856, Shanghai: Dadong shuju, 1936.

Shen Jin'ao 沈金鰲, *Fuke yuchi* 婦科玉尺 (The jade rule of medicine for women), orig. 1773, Shanghai: Kexue jishu chubanshe, 1958.

——, *Youke shimi* 幼科釋謎 (Explanations of the mysteries of medicine for infants), orig. 1773, Taibei: Wuzhou chubanshe, 1985.

Shen Youpeng 沈又彭 (zi Yaofeng), *Nüke jiyao* 女科輯要 (Essentials of medicine for women), orig. 1764, 1850 edn.

Shen Yuan 沈源, *Qizhenghui* 奇症匯 (Collection of strange disorders), orig. 1786, Beijing: Zhongyi guji chubanshe, 1981.

Shi Wen *et al.* (eds) 施雯, *Panzhuji taichan zhengzhi* 盤珠集胎產症治 (Remedies for childbirth disorders), orig. 1761, repr. in *Zhongguo yixue dacheng* 中國醫學大成, Beijing: Yuelu shushe, 1936.

Sun Simo 孫思邈, *Beiji qianjin yaofang* 備急千金要方 (Book of remedies), orig. 652, 1878 edn.

Sun Zhihong 孫志宏, *Jianming yigou* 簡明醫彀 (Concise essentials of medicine), orig. 1629, Beijing: Renmin weisheng chubanshe, 1984.

Tang Qianqing 唐千頃, *Dasheng yaozhi* 大生要旨 (Essentials on successful childbirth), orig. 1762, 1847 edn.

——, *Sanke dasheng hebi* 三科大生合璧 (Three books on successful childbirth), orig. 1762 edn.

Wan Quan 萬全, *Youke fahui* 幼科發揮 (Exposition of medicine for infants), orig. 1549, Beijing: Renmin weisheng chubanshe, 1963.

——, *Wan shi furenke* 萬氏婦人科 (Wan Quan's medicine for women), orig. 1549, Wuhan: Hubei renmin chubanshe, 1983.

——, *Yuying mijue* 育嬰秘訣 (Secrets on child-rearing), orig. 1549, repr. in *Mingdai Wan Mizhai erke quanshu* 明代萬密齋兒科全書 (The collected works on medicine for children of Wan Quan), Beijing: Zhongyi guji chubanshe, 1991.

Wang Jiamo 王嘉漢, *Taichan jicui* 胎產輯萃 (Essentials of childbirth), orig. 1745 edn.

Wang Kentang 王肯堂, *Chanbao baiwen* 產寶百問 (A hundred questions on childbirth), orig. 1559, 1602 edn.

Wang Mengying 王孟英, *Guiyanlu* 歸硯录 (Writings of Wang Mengying), orig. 1838, repr. Beijing: Zhongyi guji chubanshe, 1987.

Wang Qi 王圻 and Wang Siyi 王思義, *Sancai tuhua* 三才圖劃 (Illustrated encyclopaedia), repr. Shanghai: Shanghai guji chubanshe, 1988.

Wang Yanchang 王燕昌, *Wangshi yicun* 王氏醫存 (Medical writings of Wang Yanchang), orig. 1871, Hangzhou: Jiangsu kexue jishu chubanshe, 1983.

Wang Zhe 汪喆, *Chanke xinfa* 產科心法 (Personal experience in medicine for childbirth), orig. 1780, Hangzhou: Sansan yishe, 1924.

Weng Yuanjun 翁元鈞, *Taichan mishu* 胎產秘書 (The book of secrets on childbirth), orig. 1795, Shanghai: Huiwentang xinji shuju, 1923.

Wuji 無忌, *Baoyou xinbian* 保幼新編 (New writings on the preservation of infants), orig. 1644, Beijing: Zhongguo guji chubanshe, 1988.

Wu Qian 吳謙, *Fuke xinfa yaojue* 婦科心法要訣 (Essentials of personal experiences in medicine for women), orig. 1742, repr. in *Yizong jinjian* 醫宗金鑑 (The golden mirror of medicine), orig. 1749, Beijing: Renmin weisheng chubanshe, 1988.

——, *Jinkui yaolüe zhu* 金匱要略注 (Annotations on the Golden Chamber), orig. 1742, repr. in *Yizong jinjian* 醫宗金鑑 (The golden mirror of medicine), orig. 1749, Beijing: Renmin weisheng chubanshe, 1988.

——, *Youke zabing xinfa yaojue* 幼科雜病心法要訣 (Essentials of various medical disorders in children), orig. 1742, repr. in *Yizong jinjian* 醫宗金鑑 (The golden mirror of medicine), orig. 1749, Beijing: Renmin weisheng chubanshe, 1988.

Xia Ding 夏鼎, *Youke tiejing* 幼科鐵鏡 (Iron mirror of medicine for infants), orig. 1695, Beijing: Zhongguo shudian chubanshe, 1987.

Xiao Xun 蕭壎, *Nüke jinglun* 女科經綸 (Classified treatise in medicine for women), orig. 1684, repr. in *Zhongguo yixue dacheng*, 中國醫學大成, Beijing: Yuelu shushe, 1936.

Xiong Bolong 熊伯龍, *Wuheji* 無何集 (Philosophical writings), orig. 1794, Beijing: Zhonghua shuju, 1979.

Xu Dachun 徐大椿, *Nüke yi'an* 女科醫案 (Medical cases in medicine for women), orig. 1764, repr. in *Xu Dachun yishu quanji* 徐大椿醫書全集 (Complete medical works of Xu Dachun), Beijing: Renmin weisheng chubanshe, 1988.

——, *Nüke zhiyao* 女科旨要 (Essentials of medicine for women), orig. 1764, repr. in *Xu Dachun yishu quanji* 徐大椿醫書全集 (Complete medical works of Xu Dachun), Beijing: Renmin weisheng chubanshe, 1988.

Xu Tingzhe 許廷哲, *Baochan yaozhi* 保產要旨 (Essentials of childbirth), orig. 1806, 1898 edn.

Yan Chunxi 閻純璽, *Jingyin chanke sizhong* 精印產科四種 (Reprint of *Four books on childbirth*), orig. 1730, Shanghai: Jiangdong shuju, 1920.

——, *Taichan xinfa* 胎產心法 (Personal experience in childbirth), orig. 1730, 1824 edn.

Ye Tianshi 葉天士, *Ye Tianshi youke yi'an* 葉天士幼科醫案 (Medical cases in medicine for children of Ye Tianshi), orig. 1746, Shanghai: Shijie shuju, 1921.

Yongsitang zhuren 永思堂主人, *Taichan hebi* 胎產合璧 (Two books on childbirth), orig. 1862 edn.

Yu Qiao 俞橋, *Guangsi yaoyu* 廣嗣要語 (Important words on the spreading of offspring), orig. 1544, Shanghai: Shijie shuju, 1936.

Yu Xiangdou 余象斗, *Santai wanyong zhengzong* 三台萬用正宗 (Encyclopaedia), orig. 1599.

Yue Fujia 岳甫嘉, *Miaoyizhai yixue zhengyin zhongzi bian* 妙一齋醫學正印種子編 (Yue Fujia's writings on childbirth), orig. 1635, Beijing: Zhongyi guji chubanshe, 1986.

Yun Tieqiao 惲鐵樵, *Fuke dalüe* 婦科大略 (Outline of medicine for women), orig. 1924 edn.

Zhang Boxing 張伯行, *Zhengyi tang wenji* 正誼堂文集 (Collected works of Zhang Boxing), Shanghai: Shangwu yinshuguan, 1937.

Zhang Yaosun 張曜孫, *Chanyunji* 產孕集 (On childbirth), orig. 1830, Shanghai: Dadong shuju, 1936.

Zhao Bi 趙璧, *Shuntian yisheng pian* 順天易生篇 (Easy childbirth in accordance with Heaven), orig. 1835, 1876 edn.

Zhiyu qiaoke 芝嶼樵客, *Erke xing* 兒科醒 (Medicine for children), orig. 1813, Shanghai: Qianqingtang shuju, 1937.

Zhu Jianping *et al.* (eds) 竹劍平, *Fuke mishu bazhong* 婦科秘書八種 (Eight secret books on medicine for women), Beijing: Zhongyi guji chubanshe, 1986.

Zhulinsi sengren 竹林寺僧人, *Zhulinsi nüke erzhong* 竹林寺女科二種 (Two texts on medicine for women by the Bamboo Grove monastery), orig. 1786, Beijing: Zhongyi guji chubanshe, 1993.

Republican China

Cai Luxian 蔡陸仙, *Taichan kebing wenda* 胎產科病問答 (Questions and answers about obstetric problems), Shanghai: Huadong shuju, 1937.

Cai Yuanpei 蔡元培, 'Meiyu shishi de fangfa' 美育實施的方法 (Methods to implement beautiful births) in Cai Yuanpei, *Cai Yuanpei quanji* 蔡元培全集 (The complete works of Cai Yuanpei), Beijing: Zhonghua shuju, 1984, vol. 4, pp. 211–16.

Cao Guanlai 曹觀來, *Qingchun shengli tan* 青春生理談 (Chats about the physiology of youth), Taibei: Zhengzhong shuju, 1982 (1st edn 1936).

Chai Fuyuan 柴福沅, *Xingxue ABC* 性學 ABC (ABC of sexology), Shanghai: Shijie shuju, 1928.

Chen Changheng 陳長衡 and Zhou Jianren 周建人, *Jinhualun yu shanzhongxue* 進化論與善種學 (Evolution and eugenics), Shanghai: Shangwu yinshuguan, 1925 (1st edn 1923).

Chen Da 陳達, *Renkou wenti* 人口問題 (Population problems), Shanghai: Shangwu yinshuguan, 1934.

Chen Jianshan 陳兼善, *Taijiao* 胎教 (Foetal education), Shanghai: Shangwu yinshuguan, 1926.

Chen Shoufan 陳壽凡, *Renzhong gailiangxue* 人種改良學 (Race improvement), Shanghai: Shangwu yinshuguan, 1928 (1st edn 1919).

Chen Yinghuang 陳映璜, *Renleixue* 人類學 (Anthropology), Shanghai: Shangwu yinshuguan, 1928 (1st edn 1918).

Chen Yucang 陳雨蒼, *Renti de yanjiu* 人體的研究 (Research on the human body), Shanghai: Zhengzhong shuju, 1937.

——, *Shenghuo yu shengli* 生活與生理 (Life and physiology), Taibei: Zhengzhong shuju, 1958.

Chen Zhen 陳楨, *Putong shengwuxue* 普通生物學 (General biology), Shanghai: Shangwu yinshuguan, 1924.

Cheng Hao 程浩, *Fukexue* 婦科學 (Gynaecology), Shanghai: Shangwu yinshuguan, 1950 (9th edn, 1st edn 1939).

——, *Jiezhi shengyu wenti* 節制生育問題 (Questions about birth control), Shanghai: Yadong tushuguan, 1925.

Ding Shu'an 丁淑安 and Zhou Efen 周咢芬, *Jianyi chankexue* 簡易產科學 (Easy obstetrics), Beijing: Cicheng yinshuachang, 1948.

Ding Wenjiang 丁文江, 'Zhesixue yu pudie' 哲嗣學與譜牒 (Eugenics and clan records), *Gaizao*, 3 (1920–1), no. 4, pp. 37–44, no. 6, pp. 7–16.

Dong Zhuli 董祝釐, 'Renzhong gailiangxue zhi yanjiu fangfa' 人種改良學之研究方法 (C.B. Davenport, The research methods of the science of race improvement), *Funü zazhi* 婦女雜誌, 5, no. 12 (Dec. 1919), pp. 1–8, 6, no. 1 (Jan. 1920), pp. 6–10.

Gao Xisheng 高希聖, *Chan'er zhixian ABC* 產兒制限 ABC (ABC of birth control), Shanghai: Shijie shuju, 1929.

Ge Shaolong 戈紹龍, *Nüzi weishengxue* 女子衛生學 (Science of hygiene for women), Shanghai: Youzheng shuju, 1918.

Gong Tingzhang 宮廷璋, *Renlei yu wenhua jinbu shi* 人類與文化進步史 (History of the progress of culture and mankind), Shanghai: Shangwu yinshuguan, 1926.

Gu Mingsheng 顧鳴盛, *Fangzhong yi* 房中醫 (Medicine for the bed-chamber), Shanghai: Wenming shuju, 1916 (1930, 15th edn).

Gui Zhiliang 桂質良, *Nüren zhi yisheng* 女人之一生 (A woman's life), Peking: Zhengzhong shuju, 1936.

Guo Renji 郭人驥 and Li Renlin 酈人麟, *Nüxing yangsheng jian* 女性養生鑑 (Mirror of health for women), Shanghai: Shangwu yinshuguan, 1928 (1st edn 1922).

Hao Qinming 郝欽銘, *Yichuanxue* 遺傳學 (Genetics), Shanghai: Zhengzhong shuju, 1948.

'Haimen fu chansheng liang guaihai' 海門婦產生倆怪孩 (A woman from Haimen gives birth to two monster children), *Shenbao*, 4 April 1934, 3:9.

'Houzi you weiba renlei ye you weiba' 猴子有尾巴人類也有尾巴 (Apes have tail; man has tail too), *Dagongbao*, 9 January 1936.

Hu Buchan 胡步蟾, *Youshengxue yu renlei yichuanxue* 優生學與人類遺傳學 (Eugenics and human genetics), Shanghai: Zhengzhong shuju, 1959 (1st edn 1936).

Hu Dingan 胡定安, *Shengyu changshi* 生育常識 (Common knowledge about childbirth), Shanghai: Dadong shuju, 1933.

Hu Zhenyuan 胡珍元, *Renti de shenghuo* 人體的生活 (Life of the human body), Shanghai: Shijie shuju, 1931.

Hu Zongyuan 胡宗瑗, 'Genben gaizao renzhong zhi wenti' 根本改造人種之問題 (The problem of fundamentally reforming the race), *Funü zazhi*, 5, no. 3 (March 1919), pp. 1–5.

Hua Rucheng 華汝成, *Youshengxue ABC* 優生學 ABC (ABC of eugenics), Shanghai: Shijie shuju, 1929.

Huang Shi 黃石, 'Shenma shi taijiao' 甚麼是胎教 (What is foetal education), *Funü zazhi*, 17, no. 11 (Nov. 1930), pp. 19–28.

Jiang Xiangqing 蔣湘青, *Renti celiangxue* 人體測量學 (The science of body measurements), Shanghai: Qinfen shuju, 1935.

Jin Zizhi 金子直, *Minzu weisheng* 民族衛生 (Racial hygiene), Shanghai: Shangwu yinshuguan, 1930.

'Jinghainong chan guai'er bianti sheng baimao' 靖海農產怪兒遍體生白毛 (Monster child covered with white hair born in village of Jinghai), *Xianggang gongshang*, 8 November 1934.

'Junshao nan'er bian shaonü' 俊少男兒變少女 (A handsome boy changes into a young girl), *Gongshang ribao*, 1 May 1934, 4:3.

Kang Youwei 康有為, *Datongshu* 大同書 (One World), Beijing: Guji chubanshe, 1956.

'Kuangzhong mou shouliu bianti changmao guai xiaohai' 匡仲謀收留遍體長毛怪小孩 (Small monster child covered with long hair found in Kuangzhong), *Shenbao*, 20 September 1935.

Li Baoliang 李寶梁, *Xing de zhishi* 性的知識 (Sex knowledge), Shanghai: Zhonghua shuju, 1937.

Lin Yutang, *My country and my people*, New York: John Ray, 1935.

Liu Huru 劉虎如, *Rensheng dili gaiyao* 人生地理概要 (General principles of human geography), Shanghai: Shangwu yinshuguan, 1931.

Liu Min 劉敏, *Renleixue tixi* 人類學體系 (Anthropological systems), Shanghai: Xinken shudian, 1932.

Liu Piji 劉丕基, *Renjian wujie de shengwu* 人間誤解的生物 (Misinterpretations in everyday biology), Shanghai: Shangwu yinshuguan, 1928.

——, *Shengwu nanti jieda* 生物難題解答 (Explanations of difficult problems in biology), Shanghai: Shangwu yinshuguan, 1935.

Liu Xiong 劉雄, *Yichuan yu yousheng* 遺傳與優生 (Heredity and eugenics), Shanghai: Shangwu yinshuguan, 1926 (1st edn 1924).

'Longchuan chusheng bashiri neng yan guaiying' 龍川出生八十日能言怪嬰 (Strange infant from Longchuan can speak after eighty days), *Xianggang gongshang*, 17 Sep. 1935, 2:4.

'Meixian Lumou zhi qi yi tai san zi luodi jie neng yan' 梅縣盧謀之妻一胎三子落地皆能言 (Triplets of woman from Mei county all speak at birth), *Xianggang gongshang*, 30 Nov. 1935, 2:4.

'Mian fu sheng youjiao yinghai' 沔婦生有角嬰孩 (Woman from Mian gives birth to infant with horns), *Guangmin ribao*, 10 September 1934, 4:1.

'Nanxing bian nüxing de shiyan' 男性變女性的試驗 (Experiments in transformations of male into female), 16 December 1935, *Xinwenbao*, 4:113.

'Neifenmi de ezuo — nan bian nü yu nü bian nan' 內分泌的惡作：男變女與女變男 (The evil function of hormones and sex transformations), *Xianggang gongshang*, 2 September 1936, p. 7.

'Nongfu chan guaihai bikong zhong paixie fenzhi' 農婦產怪孩鼻孔排泄糞質 (Peasant girl gives birth to monster child which excretes through nostrils), *Xianggang gongshang*, 13 July 1935, 4:2.

'Nü hua nan shen kexueshang de jieshi' 女化男身科學上的解釋 (Scientific explanation for transformations of female into male), *Xinwenbao*, 19 August 1935, 4:13.

'Nü hua nan zhi kaozheng' 女化男之考証 (Research into transformations of female into male), *Xinwenbao*, 20 March 1935, 4:14.

Pan Guangdan 潘光旦, 'Ershi nianlai shijie zhi yousheng yundong' 二十年來世界之優生運動 (The eugenics movement in the world during the last twenty years), *Dongfang zazhi*, 22, no. 22 (Nov. 1925), pp. 60–83.

——, review of Donald Young (ed.), *The american negro*, 1928, in *The China Critic*, 28 Aug. 1930, p. 838.

——, *Youshengxue* 優生學 (Eugenics), Shanghai: Shangwu yinshuguan, 1933.

——, *Yousheng yu kangzhan* 優生與抗戰 (Eugenics and war of resistance), Shanghai: Shangwu yinshuguan, 1943.

——, 'Yousheng yu minjianzukang' 優生與民健族康 (Eugenics and racial health), *Beiping chenbao*, 3 March 1935.

——, *Zhongguo lingren xueyuan zhi yanjiu* 中國伶人血緣之研究 (Research on the blood relationship of Chinese actors), Shanghai: Shangwu yinshuguan, 1941 (2nd imp. 1987).

——, *Zhongguo zhi jiating wenti* 中國之家庭問題 (Problems of the Chinese family), Shanghai: Xinyue shuju, 1940 (1st edn 1928).

——, 'Zhongguo zhi yousheng wenti' 中國之優生問題 (China's eugenic problem), *Dongfang zazhi*, 21, no. 22 (Nov. 1924), pp. 15–32.

——, *Ziran taotai yu Zhonghua minzuxing* 自然淘汰與中華民族性 (Natural selection and the character of the Chinese race), Shanghai: Xinyue shudian, 1928.

—— (ed.), *Yousheng yuekan* 優生月刊 (Eugenics monthly), May 1931–Feb. 1932.

'Qiguai xiaotong liangge shengzhiqi zai Dadadi chenlie' 奇怪小僮兩個生殖器在大笪地陳列 (Monster child with two sexual organs exhibited on the Dada Ground), *Xianggang gongshang*, 30 May 1935, 3:2.

'Qiying yangju quan wu shen nang jida' 奇嬰陽具全無腎囊極大 (Strange infant has huge testicles but no kidneys), *Xingzhou ribao*, 6 February 1936, 3:12.

Qian Xiaoqiu 錢嘯秋, *Renzhong gailiangxue gailun* 人種改良學概論 (Introduction to the science of race improvement), Shanghai: Shenzhou guoguangshe, 1932.

'Ren bian hou zhi qiwen' 人變猴之奇聞 (Strange news about a man changing into an ape), *Beiping chenbao*, 6 June 1935.

Ru Song 如松, 'Ping youshengxue yu huanjinglun de lunzheng' 評優生學與環境論的論爭 (Review of the controversy between eugenics and environment), *Ershi shiji*, 1, no. 1 (Feb. 1931), pp. 57–124.

'Shaoxing yi laoshuang chansheng huluxing rouqiu' 紹興一老孀產生葫蘆形肉球 (Old widow from Shaoxing gives birth to flesh loaf shaped like bottle gourd), *Beiping chenbao*, 5 June 1935, p. 3.

'Sheng yi liangzhou zhi daiwei nühai' 生以兩週之帶尾女孩 (Girl with tail already two weeks old), *Zhongyang ribao*, 29 April 1936.

Shi Lu 史盧, *Yichuanxue dayi* 遺傳學大意 (Outline of heredity), Shanghai: Shenzhou guoguangshe, 1931.

'Shiri neng yan zhi guaiying' 十日能言之怪嬰 (Strange infant can speak after ten days), *Xianggang gongshang*, 11 July 1935, p. 3.

Song Jiazhao 宋嘉釗, *Taijiao* 胎教 (Foetal education), Shanghai: Zhonghua shuju, 1914.

'Songjiang Lu xing fu chansheng guaihai' 松江盧性婦產生怪孩 (Monster child born to Ms Lu in Songjiang), *Shenbao*, 14 July 1934, 3:11.

Song Mingzhi 宋銘之, *Taijiao* 胎教 (Foetal education), Shanghai: Zhonghua shuju, 1914.

Su Yizhen 蘇儀真, *Funü shengyu lun* 婦女生育論 (About women bearing children), Shanghai: Zhonghua shuju, 1922.

——, *Nüxing weisheng changshi* 女性衛生常識 (Elementary knowledge of female hygiene), Shanghai: Zhonghua shuju, 1941 (1st edn 1935).

Sun Benwen 孫本文, *Renkoulun ABC* 人口論 ABC (ABC of population theories), Shanghai: Shijie shuju, 1928.

——, 'Zai lun wenhua yu youshengxue' 再論文化與優生學 (Culture and eugenics again), *Shehui xuejie*, 1, no. 2 (Feb. 1927), pp. 1–8.

Wang Chengpin 汪誠品, *Qingchun de xingjiaoyu* 青春的性教育 (Sex education for youth), Shanghai: Xiongdi chubanshe, 1939.

Wang Chuanying (tr.) 王傳英, 'Xin taijiao' 新胎教 (New foetal education), *Funü zazhi*, 4, no. 1–2 (Jan.–Feb. 1918).

Wang Qishu 王其澍, *Yichuanxue gailun* 遺傳學概論 (Introduction to heredity), Shanghai: Shangwu yinshuguan, 1926.

Wang Yang 汪洋, *Shengyu guwen* 生育顧問 (Advice on childbirth), Shanghai: Zhongyang shuju, 1933.

Xishen (tr.) 西神, 'Renshenzhong zhi jingshen ganying' 妊娠中之精神感應 (Spiritual impressions during pregnancy), *Funü zazhi*, 2, no. 10 (Oct. 1916), pp. 13–15.

Xia Yuzhong 夏宇眾, 'Shuzhongxue yu jiaoyu' 淑種學與教育 (Eugenics and education), *Xinjiaoyu*, 2, no. 4 (Dec. 1919), pp. 395–8.

'Xiaohai you ertou, yitou hanshui, yitou qingxing' 小孩有二頭，一頭鼾睡一頭清醒 (Baby has two heads, one asleep, one awake), *Shenbao*, 23 May 1934, 3:10.

Yancheng 嵒成, 'Fatu zhi yuanyin ji qi yufang' 髮禿之原因及其預防 (The reasons and prevention of baldness), *Dongfang zazhi*, 16, no. 2 (Feb. 1919), pp. 201–2.

Yan Fu 顏復, *Yan Fu shiwen xuan* 顏復詩文選 (Selected poems and writings of Yan Fu), Beijing: Renmin wenxue chubanshe, 1959.

Yao Changxu 姚昶緒, *Taichan xuzhi* 胎產須知 (Essentials of obstetrics), Shanghai: Shangwu yinshuguan, 1929 (1st edn 1920).

'Yinyangren' 陰陽人 (Hermaphrodism), *Shenbao*, 25 February 1935, 4:16.

You Jiade 游嘉德, *Renlei qiyuan* 人類起源 (Origins of mankind), Shanghai: Shijie shuju, 1929.

'You wei renzhong yu shiren renzhong de faxian' 有尾人種與食人人種的發現 (Discovery of a race of men with tails and a race of cannibals), *Dongfang zazhi*, 26, no. 5 (March 1929), pp. 99–101.

Yu Fengbin 俞鳳賓, *Geren weisheng pian* 個人衛生篇 (Personal hygiene), Shanghai: Shangwu yinshuguan, 1931 (1st edn 1917).

Yu Jingrang 于景讓, *Renzhong gailiang* 人種改良 (Improvement of the race), Shanghai: Zhengzhong shuju, 1947 (1st edn 1936).

Zhang Jingsheng 張競生, *Mei de shehui zuzhifa* 美的社會組織法 (Plan for a beautiful society), Beijing: Beixin shuju, 1926.

Zhang Junjun 張君俊, *Minzu suzhi zhi gaizao* 民族素質之改造 (The reform of the race's quality), Shanghai: Shangwu yinshuguan, 1943.

——, *Zhongguo minzu zhi gaizao* 中國民族之改造 (The reform of the Chinese race), Shanghai: Zhonghua shuju, 1937 (1st edn 1935).

——, *Zhongguo minzu zhi gaizao, xubian* 中國民族之改造，續編 (Sequel to the reform of the Chinese race), Shanghai: Zhonghua shuju, 1936.

Zhang Ziping 張資平, *Renlei jinhualun* 人類進化論 (The theory of human evolution), Shanghai: Shangwu yinshuguan, 1930.

Zhang Zuoren 張作人, *Renlei tianyan shi* 人類天演史 (History of human evolution), Shanghai: Shangwu yinshuguan, 1930.

Zhao Shifa 趙士法, *Geren weishengxue* 個人衛生學 (Personal hygiene), Nanjing: Nanjing shudian, 1933.

'Zhongshanxian Lanbianxu faxian liangxing guaiying' 中山縣欖邊墟發現兩性怪嬰 (Infant with two sexes discovered on the market of Lanbian in Zhongshan county), *Gongshang ribao*, 2 June 1934, 2:4.

Zhou Jianren 周建人, *Lun youshengxue yu zhongzu qishi* 論優生學與種族歧視 (About eugenics and racial discrimination), Beijing: Sanlian shudian, 1950.

——, 'Shanzhongxue de lilun yu shishi' 善種學的理論與實施 (The theory of eugenics and its implementation), *Dongfang zazhi*, 18, no. 2 (Jan. 1921), pp. 56–64.

——, 'Shanzhongxue yu qi jianlizhe' 善種學與其建立者 (Eugenics and its founders), *Dongfang zazhi*, 17, no. 18 (Sept. 1920), pp. 69–75.

Zhu Haisu 朱海蕭 (ed.), *Taijiao* 胎教 (Foetal education), Shanghai: Wenye shuju, 1937.

Zhu Weiji 朱維基, *Shengwu de jinhua* 生物的進化 (Evolution of organisms), Shanghai: Yongxiang yinshuguan, 1948 (1st edn 1945).

Zhu Wenyin 朱文印, 'Taijiao yu youshengxue' 胎教與優生學 (Foetal education and eugenics), *Funü zazhi*, 17, no. 8 (Aug. 1931), pp. 11–19.

Zhu Xi 朱洗, *Cixiong zhi bian* 雌雄之變 (The changes of female and male), Shanghai: Wenhua shenghuo chubanshe, 1945.

——, *Danshengren yu renshengdan* 蛋生人與人生蛋 (The evolution of sex), Shanghai: Wenhua shenghuo chubanshe, 1939.

——, *Zhong nü qing nan* 重女輕男 (Women over men), Shanghai: Wenhua shenghuo chubanshe, 1941.

Zhu Yunping 朱雲平, *Xingjiaoyu gailun* 性教育概論 (Outline of sex education), Shanghai: Shijie shuju, 1941.

Zhu Zhenjiang 祝枕江, *Rufang ji qita* 乳房及其他 (About breasts and other things), Shanghai: Kaiming shudian, 1933.

Zhuang Weizhong 莊畏仲, *Fuying weishengxue* 婦嬰衛生學 (Hygiene for women), Nanjing: Xinyi jinxiushe, 1939.

——, *Jiankangshu wenda* 健康術問答 (Questions and answers on the art of health), Shanghai: Dahua shuju, 1934.

People's Republic of China

Ai Qionghua 艾瓊華 *et al.*, 'Xinjiang Yili wuge shaoshu minzu de jinqin jiehun' 新疆伊犁五個少數民族的近親結婚 (Consanguineous marriages among five minority nationalities in Yili, Xinjiang), *Renleixue xuebao*, 1985, no. 3, pp. 242–9.

An Hao 安好 and Kang Jindong 康金東, *Taijiao yu'er zhidao* 胎教育兒指導 (Guide to foetal education), Tianjin: Nankai daxue chubanshe, 1992.

Bakhy, Abudula, 'Tulufan shijiaoqu Weiwuerzu de jinqin jiehunlü ji yichuanxue xiaoying' 吐魯番市郊區維吾爾族的近親結婚率及遺傳學效應 (Rates of inbreeding and their genetic effects in Uyghurs of the suburbs of Turpan), *Yichuan*, 1996, no. 3, pp. 252–3.

Beijing fuchan yiyuan 北京婦產醫院 (eds), *Fuchan ji ying'er de yingyang yu baojian* 婦產及嬰兒的營養與保健 (Health protection and nutrition for pregnant women and infants), Beijing: Zhongguo shangye chubanshe, 1990.

Cao Shaoman 曹少曼, 'Chaosheng xianxiang zhenduan tai'er chunlie jixing' 超聲顯象診斷胎兒唇裂畸形 (Ultrasonic diagnosis of the harelip defect in the foetus), *Zhongguo chaosheng yixue zazhi*, 1995, no. 10, pp. 770–2.

Chai Fachen 柴法臣, 'Cong shehui xiaoyi chufa jiji kaizhan yousheng youyu gongzuo' 從社會效益出發積極開展優生優育工作 (To set up and urgently develop eugenic work for the benefit of society), *Jiankangbao*, 17 January 1986.

Chen Yandong 陳延棟, 'Tigao renkou suzhi dui kongzhi renkou shuliang de zhanlüe yiyi' 提高人口素質對控制人口數量的戰略意義 (The strategic meaning of improving the quality of the population versus limiting the quantity of the population), *Renkou yu yousheng*, 1991, no. 1, pp. 18–19.

Chen Yizhong 陳毅忠 and Hou San 侯三, *Sheng nan sheng nü youxuanfa* 生男生女優選法 (Methods to choose the sex of the baby), Wuhan: Hubei kexue jishu chubanshe, 1993.

Cheng Yufang 程玉芳, *Tai'er jixing de chaosheng zhenduan* 胎兒畸形的超聲診斷 (Ultrasonic diagnosis of foetal malformations), Beijing: Huaxia chubanshe, 1993.

Cong Li 從利, 'Yousheng zhong de "shaixuan" yu daode' 優生中的篩選與道德 (Ethics and eugenic selection), *Shandong yike daxue xuebao*, 1989, no. 2, pp. 13–14.

Dai Zhi 戴幟, *Renti zenggao de zuixin kexue jishu* 人體增高的最新科學技術 (The newest technology to increase body height), Beijing: Zhongguo yiyao keji chubanshe, 1993.

Dangdai Zhongguo de jihua shengyu shiye 當代中國的計劃生育事業 (Current family planning activities in China), Beijing: Dangdai Zhongguo chubanshe, 1992.

Deng Jungang 鄧俊剛, 'Tigao renkou zhiliang shi shidai de yaoqiu' 提高人口質量是時代的要求 (To develop the quality of the population is a requirement of our time), *Renkouxue*, 1984, no. 5, pp. 57–9.

Fang Fang 方芳, *Yousheng yu youyu* 優生與優育 (Eugenics and quality childbirth), Beijing: Renmin chubanshe, 1991.

Fang Xiao 方曉, 'Hewei renkou zhiliang?' 何謂人口質量 (What is called population quality?), *Beifang dili jiaoxue*, Feb. 1986.

Fei Xiaotong 費孝通, 'Zhongguo yao zuohao liangjian renkou dashi' 中國要作好兩間人口大事 (China needs to complete two important demographic tasks), *Zhongguo jihua shengyubao*, 9 Oct. 1987, p. 3.

Fu Caiying 傅才英, *Sheng er yu nü sanbai wen* 生兒育女三百問 (Three hundred questions on childbirth and child rearing), Beijing: Jindun chubanshe, 1987 (13th repr. 1994).

Gao Jinsheng 高錦聲, 'Yichuanbing shi yousheng de dadi' 遺傳病是優生的大敵 (Hereditary diseases are the great enemy of eugenic births), *Renkouxue*, 1985, no. 4, pp. 43–4.

Ge Ming 葛明, 'Youshengxue' 優生學 (Eugenics), *Wenhuibao*, 23 July 1984, p. 3.

Gu Huayun (ed.) 谷華運, *Zhongguoren peitai fayu shixu he jitai yufang* 中國人胚胎發育時序和畸胎預防 (The development of the embryo in Chinese people and the prevention of malformations), Shanghai: Yike daxue chubanshe, 1993.

Hu Jize 胡紀澤, 'Yao dong yidian youshengxue (jieshao Pan Guangdan de *Yousheng yuanli*)' 要懂一點優生學（介紹潘光旦的優生原理）(We should understand some eugenics: Introducing Pan Guangdan's *Eugenic principles*), *Renkouxue*, 1986, no. 3, pp. 74–6.

Hu Tingyi (ed.) 胡廷溢, *Xing shenghuo zixun* 性生活咨詢 (Advice on sex life), Nanchang: Jiangxi kexue jishu chubanshe, 1990.

Hu Weiqin 胡惟勤, 'Jingshen bingren de hunyin wenti' 精神病人的婚姻問題 (The question of marriage for mentally sick people), *Renkou yu yousheng*, 1988, no. 1, p. 11.

Huang Jianmin 黃建民, 'Fandui zaochu xin renzhong' 反對造出新人種 (Against the making of a new race), *Jiankang shijie*, 1996, no. 6, pp. 38–9.

Jiang Jianhong 姜建鴻, '"Kexue youshengshu" bing bu kexue' 科學優生術并不科學 ('Scientific art of eugenics' is not scientific at all), *Renkou yu yousheng*, 1990, no. 1, p. 7.

Li Chonggao 李崇高, 'Youshengxue youguan wenti de taolun' 優生學有關問題的討論 (A discussion of problems regarding eugenics), *Xibei renkou*, 1985, no. 2, pp. 38–42.

Li Song 李松 and Qiang Aixi 強艾希, *Chusheng quexian zhenduan tupu* 出生缺陷診斷圖譜 (Illustrations for the diagnosis of malformations at birth), Beijing: Beijing yike daxue chubanshe, 1992.

Li Zhigui 李之桂 and Meng Xianwen 孟憲文, *Taijiao* 胎教 (Foetal education), Beijing: Kexue jishu chubanshe, 1991 (2nd repr. 1992).

Li Zi 李子, *Taijiao* 胎教 (Foetal education), Xi'an: Shanxi renmin chubanshe, 1986.

Lian Xiaohua 連孝華, 'Zeshi shouyun hua yousheng' 擇時受孕話優生 (Eugenics and the choice of the time for conception), *Renkou yu yousheng*, 1992, no. 3, p. 6.

Liao Zhifang 廖之芳 and Zhong Xin 鍾心, *Renti zenggao de mijue* 人體增高的秘訣 (Secrets to increase body height), Guangxi kexue jishu chubanshe, 1991.

Liu Chaoyu 劉朝裕, *Yichuan yu chusheng quexian zonghezheng* 遺傳與出生缺陷綜合症 (Heredity and malformations), Chengdu: Sichuan kexue jishu chubanshe, 1992.

Liu Jianli 劉建立 et al., *Nüxing qingchunqi baojian 170 wen* 女性青春期保健 170 問 (170 questions about health during the period of female puberty), Beijing: Jindun chubanshe, 1992 (3rd repr. 1994).

Liu Jinxiang 劉金香, 'Ping Pan Guangdan de *Yousheng gailun*' 評潘光旦的優生概論 (A review of Pan Guangdan's *Introduction to eugenics*), *Yichuan*, 1982, no. 3, pp. 39–40.

Liu Qi 劉奇, 'Tai'er xingbie jianding jishu yingyong de lunli daode wenti' 胎兒性別鑒定技術應用的倫理道德問題 (Ethical questions on the use of tests for prenatal sex determination), *Zhongguo yixue lunlixue*, 1995, no. 2, pp. 46–7.

Liu Qingxian 劉慶憲, 'Kua shiji de shengzhi geming' 跨世紀的生殖革命 (A reproductive revolution which straddles the next century), *Yixue yu zhexue*, 1994, no. 4, pp. 33–4.

Liu Shijing 劉士敬 et al., 'Beijing shi 360 ming butong renqun dui you quexian xinsheng'er chuli yijian de diaocha yu fenxi' 北京市360名不同人群對有缺陷新生兒處理意見調查與分析 (Investigation and analysis of the attitudes towards the treatment of disabled neonates of 360 people of different social backgrounds in Beijing municipality), *Zhongguo yixue lunlixue*, 1990, no, 10, pp. 29–30.

Liu Zhengxue 劉正學, *Zenyang shengge guai wawa* 怎樣生個乖娃娃 (How to give birth to a well-behaved baby), Chengdu: Sichuan kexue jishu chubanshe, 1991.

Luo Hong 羅虹 and Jiang Chaoguǎng 江朝光, *Taijiao yu yousheng 200 wen* 胎教與優生200問 (200 questions about foetal education and superior birth), Beijing: Jindun chubanshe, 1992 (5th repr. 1994).

Mu Guangzong 穆光宗, 'Lun Zhongguo renkou de suzhi kongzhi: Guanyu Zhonghua minzu weilai de shehuixue sikao' 論中國人口的素質控制：關於中華民族未來的社會學思考 (The control of the quality of China's population: Sociological considerations about the future of the Chinese nation), *Renkouxue*, 1991, no. 4, pp. 73–80.

Na Li 娜麗, *Taijiao fangfa* 胎教方法 (Methods of foetal education), Beijing: Zhongyang minzu xueyuan chubanshe, 1988.

Pan Ronghua 潘榮華 and Zhou Xiaojun 周曉鈞, '448 ren dui quexian xinsheng'er de chuli diaocha baogao' 448人對缺陷新生兒的處理調查報告 (Report on an investigation of 448 persons' attitudes towards the treatment of disabled neonates), *Yixue yu zhexue*, 1988, no. 3, pp. 28–30.

Qiu Jinghua 邱景華, 'Ruozhi ertong de kangfu xunlian' 弱智兒僮的康復訓練 (Rehabilitation exercices for mildly retarded children), *Jiankang shijie*, 1996, no. 6, pp. 16–17.

Qiu Renzong 邱仁宗, 'Dui zhili yanzhong dixiazhe shixing jueyu de lunlixue wenti' 對智力嚴重低下者施行絕育的倫理學問題 (Some ethical questions about the sterilisation of severely retarded people), *Zhongguo yixue lunlixue*, 1992, no. 1, pp. 10–15.

Qu Jianding 屈堅定, 'Cong ziran xuanze dao rengong xuanze: tan renkou shenti suzhi he yichuan jiyin' 從自然選擇到人工選擇：談人口身體素質和遺傳基因 (From natural selection to artificial selection: About inherited genes and the physical quality of the population), repr. in *Renkouxue*, 1987, no. 2, pp. 76–8.

Quan Wenfu 權文富 and Zhang De'an 張德安, 'DNA xinxi yu yousheng' DNA信息與優生 (Eugenics and news about DNA), *Renkou xuekan*, 1983, no. 3, pp. 63–65.

'Renkou zhiliang weiji' 人口質量危機 (The crisis of population quality), *Gongrenbao*, 29 April 1989.

Shen Huiyun 沈惠雲, 'Wo chang de "taijiao" shi' 我廠的胎教室 (Our factory's 'foetal education' office), *Renkou yu yousheng*, 1995, no. 47, p. 9.

Song Weimin 宋為民 and Lu Yuelian 陸月蓮, *Renti shengwuzhong qutan* 人體生物鍾趣談 (Interesting stories about the human body's biological clock), Shanghai: Zhongyi xueyuan chubanshe, 1990.

——, *Shengwuzhong yangsheng* 生物鍾養生 (The biological clock and the nourishment of life), Tianjin: Tianjin kexue jishu chubanshe, 1990.

Su Liwen 蘇麗雯 and Lu Qiyi 路齊一, *Shengli weisheng zhishi* 生理衛生知識 (Knowledge of physiological hygiene), Beijing: Zhongguo chubanshe, 1989.

Su Ping 蘇蘋 and Hou Dongmin 侯東民, *Youshengxue gailun* 優生學概論 (Introduction to eugenics), Beijing: Renmin daxue chubanshe, 1994.

Sun Nianhu 孫念怙, *Yichuanxing jibing de chanqian zhenduan* 遺傳性疾病的產前診斷 (The diagnosis of hereditary malformations before birth), Beijing: Renmin weisheng chubanshe, 1983.

Sun Puquan 孫溥泉, *Renti qiwen lu* 人體奇聞錄 (Record of fantastic stories about the human body), Zhengzhou: Tianze chubanshe, 1989.

Taijiao yingyou'er zaoqi jiaoyu sibai wen 胎教嬰幼兒早期教育四百問 (Four hundred questions about the foetal education and the raising of infants), Beijing: Haiyang chubanshe, 1994.

Tao Kan 陶侃, 'Fushu diqu yuanhe ruozhi ertong yuelai yueduo' 富庶地區緣何弱智兒僮越來越多 (Why retarded children are on the increase in rich and populous regions), *Renkou yu yousheng*, 1996, no. 4, p. 3.

'Tigao renkou suzhi de guanjian zai nongcun' 提高人口素質的關鍵在農村 (The key to improving the quality of the population lies in the countryside), *Renkou yu yousheng*, 1993, no. 1, pp. 24–5.

Tian Lihong 田麗紅, 'Lüe lun rencai, zhili yu yousheng' 略論人才，智力與優生 (Brief comments about talent, intelligence and eugenics), *Huazhong shifan daxue xuebao*, 1991, no. 3, pp. 106–7.

'Tuixing yousheng, zhenxing Zhonghua' 推行優生，振興中華 (To implement eugenics and to develop the nation), *Renkou yu jingji*, 25 Jan. 1984.

Wan Fang 萬鈁, *Youshengxue* 優生學 (Eugenics), Beijing: Shifan daxue chubanshe, 1994.

Wang Huiren *et al.* 王惠人, *Shenjing shuairuo fangzhi 100 wen* 神經衰弱防治100問 (100 questions about the treatment of neurasthenia), Beijing: Jindun chubanshe, 1992 (2nd repr. 1993).

Wang Man 王曼 *et al.* (eds), *Shiyong fuchanke shouce* 實用婦產科手冊 (Handbook of applied obstetrics), Zhejiang kexue jishu chubanshe, 1989.

Wang Ping (tr.) 王蘋, *Zenyang sheng congming jiankang de haizi: taijiao* 怎樣生聰明健康的孩子：胎教 (How to give birth to an intelligent and healthy child: Foetal education), Beijing: Kexue jishu wenxian chubanshe, 1993.

Wang Ruiduo 王瑞多, 'Jiantan renkou zhiliang yu shehui fazhan de guanxi' 簡談人口質量與社會發展的關系 (Brief discussion about the relationship between population quality and social development), *Renkouxue*, 1987, no. 1, p. 110.

Wang Ruizi 王瑞梓, 'Zhongguo renkou wenti de zhongdian zai nongcun' 中國人口問題的重點在農村 (The core of demographic problems is in the countryside), *Renkou yu yousheng*, 1991, no. 2, pp. 3–4.

Wang Ruogu 王若谷, "Wen Xinjiapo xin renkou zhengce you gan' 聞新加坡新人口政策有感 (The population policy in Singapore), *Renkou yu yousheng*, 1992, no. 4, p. 26.

Wang Xiangchu 王祥初, 'Ye lun dui yanzhong xiantian quexian binghuan er de sheqi' 也論對嚴重先天缺陷病患兒的捨棄 (Again about the abandonment of severely congenitally handicapped neonates), *Yixue yu zhexue*, 1985, no. 11, pp. 53–55.

Wang Yijiong 王義炯, *Renti zhi mi* 人體之謎 (Mysteries of the human body), Shanghai: Wenhui chubanshe, 1988.

Wen Ming 聞明, *Xin shenghuo de jin yaoshi* 新生活的金鑰匙 (The golden key to a new life), Taiyuan: Shanxi jingji chubanshe, 1994.

Weng Xiayun 翁霞雲, *Jihua shengyu yu yousheng 200 wen* 計劃生育與優生200問 (200 questions about birth control and eugenics), Beijing: Jindun chubanshe, 1992.

Wu Shuming 吳樹明, 'Xiandai shenghuo yu yousheng' 現代生活與優生 (Contemporary life and eugenics), *Renkou yu yousheng*, 1993, no. 6, p. 10.

Wu Zhongguan 吳忠觀, 'Shilun renkou zhiliang' 試論人口質量 (About population quality), *Renkou yu jingji*, 1984, no. 6, pp. 3–6.

Wu Zhangming *et al.* 吳章明, *Hunqian hunhou weisheng sanbai wen* 婚前婚後衛生三百問 (Three hundred questions about hygiene before and after marriage), Fuzhou: Fujian kexue jishu chubanshe, 1987 (11th repr. 1992).

Xiao Hua 孝華, 'Jixing hunyin jixing er' 畸形婚姻畸形兒 (Freak marriage leads to freak child), *Renkou yu yousheng*, 1992, no. 2, p. 10.

Xin Xiang 昕祥, 'Youshengxue gaishu' 優生學概述 (Outline of eugenics), *Renkouxue*, 1985, no. 11, p. 14.

Xing Shumin 邢淑敏, *Yunchanfu baojian 300 wen* 孕產婦保健300問 (Three hundred questions on health during pregnancy), Beijing: Jindun chubanshe, 1991 (10th repr. 1994).

Xu Bin 徐斌, *Xing shenghuo yehua* 性生活夜話 (Evening talks about sex life), Changchun: Jilin kexue jishu chubanshe, 1989 (4th repr. 1993).

Xu Gailing 許改玲, 'Sichuan shouci renkou suzhi yantaohui guandian zongshu' 四川首次人口素質研討會觀點綜述 (Abstract of the standpoint of Sichuan province's first meeting to discuss population quality), *Shehui kexue yanjiu*, 1986, no. 6, pp. 125–6.

Xu Yi 徐藝, 'Tigao renkou suzhi, shiying sidahua jianshe xuyao' 提高人口素質，適應四大化建設須要 (To improve the quality of the population is a requirement for the Four Modernizations), *Guizhou ribao*, 27 Jan. 1986.

Yan Renying 嚴仁英 and Lin Guimei 林佳楣, *Shiyong yousheng shouce* 實用優生手冊 (Handbook of applied eugenics), Beijing: Renmin weisheng chubanshe, 1992.

Yang Nairong 楊乃榮, 'Bu ying sheqi yanzhong xiantian quexian binghuan er' 不應捨棄嚴重先天缺陷病患兒 (Against the abandonment of severely congenitally handicapped neonates), *Yixue yu zhexue*, 1985, no. 6, p. 49.

Yang Xiuting 楊秀婷 *et al.* (eds), *Taijiao, weiyang, baojian* 胎教，喂養，保健 (Foetal education, child feeding and health protection), Harbin: Heilongjiang jiaoyu chubanshe, 1988.

Ye Gongshao 葉恭紹 *et al.* , *Ertong, shaonian xing zhishi qimeng* 兒僮，少年性知識啟蒙 (Rudimentary sex knowledge for children and young people), Shenyang: Liaoning kexue jishu chubanshe, 1991.

Ye Wenhu 葉文虎 and Zhu Wenhua 朱文華, *Hunyin yu yousheng* 婚姻與優生 (Marriage and eugenics), Hefei: Anhui kexue jishu chubanshe, 1983 (4th repr. 1990).

Ying Wenhui 應文輝, 'Yingxiang yousheng de qi da huohai' 影響優生的七大禍害 (The seven great dangers to eugenics), *Renkou yu yousheng*, 1992, no. 1, p. 8.

Yousheng xuzhi 優生須知 (Essentials of eugenics), Beijing: Renmin weisheng chubanshe, 1981.

Yu Guanjian 余關鍵, 'Yousheng xuanchuan ying zhongshi kexuexing' 優生宣傳應重視科學性 (Eugenic propaganda should pay more attention to scientific credibility), *Renkou yu yousheng*, 1994, no. 2, p. 6.

Yuan Huarong 原華榮, 'Lun yousi de shehui jingji yiyi he daode jiazhi' 論優死的社會經濟意義和道德價值 (About the social and economic meaning of euthanasia and its moral value), *Renkou yanjiu*, 1990, no. 4.

Zhang Chunqing 張春卿 and Liu Guirong 劉桂榮, 'Kedingbing huanzhe de hunyu yu yousheng lifa' 克汀病患者的婚育與優生立法 (Cretinism and marriage in the light of eugenic legislation), *Yixue yu zhexue*, 1991, no. 8, pp. 44–5.

Zhang Juan 張娟 and Qin Chao 秦潮, '296 li shangcan qi'er de shengming lunlixue fenxi' 296例傷殘棄兒的生命倫理學分析 (Bioethical analysis on 296 cases of abandoned children with disabilities), *Yixue yu zhexue*, 1989, no. 8, pp. 30–2.

Zhang Shaoying 張少英, *Yixue yichuanxue gaiyao* 醫學遺傳學概要 (Basics of medical genetics), Harbin: Heilongjiang kexue jishu chubanshe, 1985.

Zhang Tianjin 張天金, *Fuqi shenghuo 365* 夫妻生活365 (365 questions about conjugal life), Fuzhou: Fuzhou kexue jishu chubanshe, 1988.

Zhang Wanying 張婉英, 'Zhongguo gudairen tan yousheng' 中國古代人談優生 (Eugenics in ancient China), *Jiankangbao: Jihua shengyuban*, 10 April 1987, p. 3.

Zhang Yanlong 張彥龍, 'Jingzi, yousheng zhi ben' 精子，優生之本 (Semen, a eugenic capital), *Renkou yu yousheng*, 1994, no. 6, p. 5.

Zhao Gongmin 趙功民, *Yichuanxue yu shehui* 遺傳學與社會 (Genetics and society), Shenyang: Liaoning renmin chubanshe, 1986.

'Zhejiang sheng yousheng baojian tiaoli' 浙江省優生保健條理 (Zhejiang province's regulations in eugenics and the protection of health), *Renkou yu yousheng*, 1992, no. 3, p. 5.

Zheng Fozhou 鄭佛州 *et al.*, *Xing chuanbo jibing fangzhi 100 wen* 性傳播疾病防治 100 問 (100 questions about the treatment of sexually transmitted diseases), Beijing: Jindun chubanshe, 1990 (6th repr. 1993).

Zheng Richang 鄭日昌 *et al.* (eds), *Xing xinli zixun* 性心理咨詢 (Advice on the psychology of sex), Nanchang: Jiangxi kexue jishu chubanshe, 1990.

Zheng Guizhen 鄭規真, 'Tigao renkou zhiliang he shixian shehuizhuyi xiandaihua' 提高人口質量和施現社會主義現代化 (The improvement of the population and the implementation of socialist modernisation), *Renkouxue*, 1986, no. 5, pp. 108–110.

Zhongguo kexue puji ji gongzuo bu *et al.* (eds) 中國科學普及及工作部, *Yousheng yu ying'er baojian* 優生與嬰兒保健 (Eugenics and health protection for infants), Beijing: Kexue puji chubanshe, 1990.

'Zhongguo renkou zhiliang taolunhui zai Beijing zhaokai' 中國人口質量討論會在北京召開 (Opening of a conference in Beijing on the quality of the Chinese population), *Renkou xuekan*, 1984, no. 6, p. 56.

'Zhonghua renmin gongheguo muying baojian fa' 中華人民共和國母嬰保健法 (The People's Republic of China's maternal and infant health law), *Zhonghua renmin gongheguo quanguo renmin daibiao dahui changwu weiyuanhui gongbao*, 1994, no. 7, pp. 3–8.

Zhou Haobai 周皓白, *Jitai zongheng tan* 畸胎縱橫談 (Talks about malformations), Hangzhou: Jiangsu kexue jishu chubanshe, 1985.

Zhou Xianzhi 周顯志 and Li Xiaowei 李小衛, 'Shengming zhiliang dilie xinsheng'er "yousi" tantao' 生命質量低劣新生兒優死探討 (Discussion of euthanasia of infants of inferior quality), *Renkou yanjiu*, 1995, no. 3, pp. 58–61.

Zhou Xiaozheng 周孝正, 'Ershiyi shiji de Zhongguo renkou yu yousheng' 二十一世紀的中國人口與優生 (The Chinese population and eugenics in the twenty-first century), *Renkouxue*, 1988, no. 4, pp. 81–6.

Zhu Hong 朱宏, 'Lianyin fanwei yu renkou suzhi' 聯姻範圍與人口素質 (The scope of marriage and population quality), *Zhong Gong*

Zhejiang Shengwei Dangxiao (Communist Party of China's Zhejiang Provincial Party Committee School), March 1990, pp. 29–35, reprinted in *Renkouxue*, 1990, no. 5, pp. 96–100.

Zou Guangzhong 鄒光忠, *Renti zhi mi* 人體之謎 (The mysteries of the human body), Beijing: Xinhua chubanshe, 1989.

SECONDARY SOURCES

Adams, Mark B., 'Eugenics in Russia, 1900–1940' in Mark B. Adams (ed.), *The wellborn science: Eugenics in Germany, France, Brazil and Russia*, Oxford University Press, 1990, pp. 110–216.

———, *The wellborn science: Eugenics in Germany, France, Brazil and Russia*, Oxford University Press, 1990.

Baines, Barry and David Bloor, 'Relativism, rationalism and the sociology of knowledge', Martin Hollis and Steven Lukes (eds), *Rationality and relativism*, Oxford: Blackwell, 1982, pp. 21–47.

Bakken, Børge, 'Modernizing morality? Paradoxes of socialization in China during the 1980s', *East Asian History*, no. 2 (Dec. 1991), pp. 125–41.

Banister, Judith, *China's changing population*, Stanford University Press, 1987.

Barkan, Elazar, *The retreat of scientific racism: Changing concepts of race in Britain and the United States between the two world wars*, Cambridge University Press, 1992.

Beattie, Hilary J., *Land and lineage in China: A study of T'ung-ch'eng County, Anhwei, in the Ming and Ch'ing dynasties*, Cambridge University Press, 1979.

Benedict, Carol, 'Chinese police campaigns against persons with leprosy, 1934–37', paper presented at the Annual Meeting of the Association of Asian Studies, Chicago, 14–16 March 1996.

Biervliet, H., 'Biologisme, racisme en eugenetiek in de antropologie en sociologie van de jaren dertig' in F. Bovenkerk *et al.* (eds), *Toen en thans. De sociale wetenschappen in de jaren dertig en nu*, Baarn: Ambo, 1978, pp. 208–35.

Bogdan, Robert, *Freak show: Presenting human oddities for amusement and profit*, University of Chicago Press, 1988.

Bond, D.F., '"Distrust" of imagination in English neoclassicism', *Philological Quarterly*, no. 14 (1937), pp. 54–69.

———, 'The neoclassical psychology of the imagination', *English Literature and History*, no. 4 (1937), pp. 245–64.

Bonniol, Jean-Luc and Pascale Gleize, 'Penser l'hérédité', *Ethnologie Française*, 24, no. 1 (Jan.–March 1994), pp. 5–10.

Borchard, Dagmar, 'Aus einem Melonenkern entsteht eine Melone. Gesetzliche Rahmenbedingungen der Eugenik', *Das Neue China*, 1994, no. 4, pp. 25–7.

——, 'VR China. Neue Vorschriften zur Kontrolle der Eheregistrierung', *Das Standesamt*, 49, no. 2 (Sept. 1996), pp. 275–80.

Borei, Dorothy V., 'Eccentricity and dissent: The case of Kung Tzu-chen', *Ch'ing-shi wen-t'i*, 3, no. 4 (Dec. 1975), pp. 50–62.

Borges, Dain, '"Puffy, ugly, slothful and inert": Degeneration in Brazilian social thought, 1880–1940', *Journal of Latin American Studies*, 25 (1993), pp. 235–56.

Boucé, Paul-Gabriel, 'Imagination, pregnant women, and monsters in eighteenth-century England and France' in G.S. Rousseau and Roy Porter (eds), *Sexual underworlds of the Enlightement*, Manchester University Press, 1987, pp. 87–100.

Bowler, P.J., *Evolution: The history of an idea*, Berkeley: University of California Press, 1984.

——, *The non-Darwinian revolution: Reinterpreting a historical myth*, Baltimore: Johns Hopkins University Press, 1988.

Braun, Christina von, 'Männliche Hysterie, Weibliche Askese: Zum Paradigmenwechsel in den Geschlechterrollen' in Karin Rick (ed.), *Das Sexuelle, die Frauen und die Kunst*, Tübingen, no date.

Broberg, Gunnar and Nils Roll-Hansen (eds), *Eugenics and the welfare state: Sterilization policy in Denmark, Sweden, Norway, and Finland*, East Lansing: Michigan State University Press, 1996.

Brokaw, Cynthia, *The ledgers of merit and demerit: Social change and moral order in late imperial China*, Princeton University Press, 1991.

Burleigh, Michael and Wolfgang Wippermann, *The racial state: Germany 1933–1945*, Cambridge University Press, 1991.

Canguilhem, Georges, 'La monstruosité et le monstrueux' in *La connaissance de la vie*, Paris: Vrin, 1992, pp. 171–84.

Carol, Anne, *Histoire de l'eugénisme en France. Les médecins et la procréation, XIXe-XXe siècle*, Paris: Seuil, 1995.

Cass, Victoria, 'Female healers in the Ming and the Lodge of Ritual and Ceremony', *Journal of the American Oriental Society*, 106, no. 1 (Jan.–March 1986), pp. 233–40.

Céard, Jean, *La nature et les prodiges*, Geneva: Droz, 1977.

Chee, Heng Leng and Chee Khoon (eds), *Designer genes: I.Q., ideology and biology*, Petaling Jaya: Institute for Social Analysis, 1984.

Chow, Kai-wing, *The rise of Confucian ritualism in late imperial China: Ethics, Classics, and lineage discourse*, Stanford University Press, 1994.

Cleminson, Richard, 'Eugenics by name or nature? The Spanish anarchist sex reform of the 1930s', *History of European Ideas*, 18 (1994), pp. 729–40.

Croll, Elisabeth J., 'A commentary on the new draft law on eugenics and health protection', *China Information*, 8, no. 3 (winter 1993–4), pp. 32–7.

Darmon, Pierre, *Le mythe de la procréation à l'âge baroque*, Paris: Seuil, 1981.

Digby, Anne and David Wright, *From idiocy to mental deficiency: Historical perspectives on people with learning disabilities*, London: Routledge, 1996.

Dikötter, Frank (ed.), *The construction of racial identities in China and Japan: Historical and contemporary perspectives*, London: C. Hurst; Honolulu: University of Hawaii Press; Sydney: Geo. Allen and Unwin, 1997.

——, 'Death by design: Euthanasia in China' (forthcoming).

——, *The discourse of race in modern China*, London: C. Hurst, Stanford University Press, Hong Kong University Press, 1992.

——, 'Eugenics in Republican China', *Republican China*, 15, no. 1 (Nov. 1989), pp. 1–18.

——, 'Hairy barbarians, furry primates and wild men: Medical science and cultural representations of hair in China' in Alf Hiltebeitel and Barbara Miller (eds), *Hair in Asian cultures: Context and change*, Albany: State University of New York Press, 1998, pp. 51–74.

——, 'A history of sexually transmitted diseases in China' in Scott Bamber, Milton Lewis and Michael Waugh (eds), *Sex, disease, and society: A comparative history of sexually transmitted diseases and HIV/AIDS in Asia and the Pacific*, Westport, CT: Greenwood Press, 1997, pp. 67–84.

——, 'The limits of benevolence: Wang Shiduo (1802–1889) and population control', *Bulletin of the School of Oriental and African Studies*, 55, no. 1 (Feb. 1992), pp. 110–15.

——, 'Race culture: Recent perspectives on the history of eugenics', *American Historical Review*, 103, no. 2 (April 1998), pp. 467–78.

——, 'Reading the body: Genetic knowledge and social marginalisation in the PRC', *China Information*, 12, no. 4 (Spring 1998).

——, *Sex, culture and modernity in China: Medical science and the construction of sexual identities in the early Republican period*, London: C. Hurst; Honolulu: University of Hawaii Press; Hong Kong University Press, 1995.

——, 'Sexualité, discipline et modernité en Chine', *Equinoxe. Déviances, intolérances et normes*, no. 13 (April 1994), 171–83.

Dubinin, N., 'Nasledovanie biologicheskoe i sotsial'noe', *Kommunist*, 11 (July 1980), pp. 62–74.

Duvernay-Bolens, Jacqueline, 'Un trickster chez les naturalistes. La notion d'hybride', *Ethnologie Française*, 23, no. 1 (Jan.–March 1993), pp. 142–52.

Ehrenström, Philippe, 'Stérilisation opératoire et maladie mentale. Une étude de cas', *Gesnerus*, 48 (1991), pp. 503–16.

Engell, James, *The creative imagination: Enlightenment to Romanticism*, Cambridge, MA: Harvard University Press, 1981.

Evans, Harriet, 'Defining difference: The "scientific" construction of gender and sexuality in the People's Republic of China', *Signs*, 20, no. 2 (Winter 1995), pp. 357–94.

——, *Women and sexuality in China*, Cambridge: Polity, 1997.

Faden, Ruth R. *et al.*, 'Prenatal screening and pregnant women's attitudes toward the abortion of defective fetuses', *American Journal of Public Health*, 77 (Feb. 1987), pp. 1–3.

Fan Shuzhi 樊樹志, *Ming Qing Jiangnan shizhen tanwei* 明清江南市鎮探微 (Studies on the cities of Jiangnan in the Ming and Qing), Shanghai: Fudan daxue chubanshe, 1990.

Fan Xingzhun 范行准, *Zhongguo yixue shilüe* 中國醫學史略 (Essentials of history of Chinese medicine), Beijing: Zhongyi guji chubanshe, 1986.

Field, Catherine, 'Scandal of China's orphanages: Medical staff sentence thousands of "troublesome and unattractive" children to death by starvation', *The Observer*, 7 January 1996, p. 19.

Fischer, Jean-Louis, 'Hérédité et tératologie, 1860–1920' in Claude Bénichou (ed.), *L'ordre des caractères. Aspects de l'hérédité dans l'histoire des sciences de l'homme*, Paris: Vrin, 1989, pp. 95–118.

——, *Monstres. Histoire du corps et de ses défauts*, Paris: Syros, 1992.

Foucault, Michel (ed.), *Herculine Barbin*, Brighton: Harvester Press, 1980.

Furth, Charlotte, 'Androgynous males and deficient females: Biology and gender boundaries in sixteenth- and seventeenth-century China', *Late Imperial China*, 9, no. 2 (Dec. 1988), pp. 1–31.

——, 'Blood, body and gender: Medical images of the female condition in China, 1600–1850', *Chinese Science*, 7 (Dec. 1986), pp. 43–66.

——, 'Concepts of pregnancy, childbirth, and infancy in Ch'ing dynasty China', *Journal of Asian Studies*, 46, no. 1 (Feb. 1987), pp. 7–35.

——, 'Talk on Ming-Qing medicine and the construction of gender', paper presented at the Institute of History and Philosophy, Taibei, 26 November 1992.

—— and Ch'en Shu-yueh, 'Chinese medicine and the anthropology of menstruation in contemporary Taiwan', *Medical Anthropology Quarterly*, 6, no. 1 (March 1992), pp. 27–48.

Gao Yuan, *Born red: A chronicle of the Cultural Revolution*, Stanford University Press, 1987.

Gilman, Sander L., *Disease and representation: Images of illness from madness to AIDS*, Ithaca, NY: Cornell University Press, 1988.

Gladney, Dru C., *Muslim Chinese: Ethnic nationalism in the People's Republic*, Cambridge, MA: Harvard University Press, 1996.

Gleize, Pascale, 'L'hérédité hors du champ scientifique', *Ethnologie Française*, 24, no. 1 (Jan.–March 1994), pp. 10–24.

Gould, Stephen Jay, *Ontogeny and phylogeny*, Cambridge, MA: Harvard University Press, 1977.

Greenhalgh, Susan, 'State society links: Political dimensions of population policies and programs, with special reference to China', *Working Paper 18*, New York: Population Council, 1990.

Gulik, Robert Hans van, *Sexual life in ancient China*, Leiden: E.J. Brill, 1974.

Guo Junshuang 郭君雙 and Tian Daihua 田代華, 'Yan Chunxi yu Taichan xinfa' 閻純璽與胎產心法 (Yan Chunxi and his book on obstetrics), *Zhonghua yishi zazhi*, 1990, 20, no. 3, pp. 180–3.

Hall, Marie Boas, *All scientists now: The Royal Society in the nineteenth century*, Cambridge University Press, 1984.

Handlin, Joanna F., *Action in late Ming thought: The reorientation of Lü K'un and other scholar-officials*, Berkeley: University of California Press, 1983.

Harding, Harry, 'The Cultural Revolution: China in turmoil, 1966–1969' in Roderick MacFarquhar and John K. Fairbank (eds), *The Cambridge history of China*, vol. 15: *The People's Republic*, part 2: *Revolutions within the Chinese revolution, 1966–1982*, Cambridge University Press, 1991, pp. 107–217.

Harrell, Stevan, 'The rich get children: Segmentation, stratification, and population in three Chekiang lineages, 1550–1850' in Susan B. Hanley and Arthur P. Wolf, *Family and population in East Asian history*, Stanford University Press, 1985, pp. 81–109.

He Zhongjun 和中浚, 'Wan Qing Sichuan puji leiyizhu de chansheng he yingxiang' 晚清四川普及類醫著的產生和影響 (The production and influence of medical books of vulgarisation in Sichuan during the late Qing), *Zhonghua yishi zazhi*, 1994, 24, no. 1, pp. 20–2.

Henderson, John B., *The development and decline of Chinese cosmology*, New York: Columbia University Press, 1984.

Heyck, T.W., *The transformation of intellectual life in Victorian England*, London: Croom Helm, 1982.

Ho Ping-ti, *The ladder of success in imperial China: Aspects of social mobility, 1368–1911*, New York: Da Capo Press, 1976.

——, *Studies on the population of China, 1368–1953*, Cambridge, MA: Harvard University Press, 1959.

Howard, Martin, *Victorian grotesque: An illustrated excursion into medical curiosities, freaks and abnormalities, principally of the Victorian age*, London: Jupiter, 1977.

Hsiao Kung-chuan, *Rural China: Imperial control in the nineteenth century*, Seattle: University of Washington Press, 1967.

Hsiung Ping-chen 熊秉真, 'Constructed emotions: The bond between mothers and sons', *Late Imperial China*, 15, no. 1 (June 1994), pp. 87–117.

——, 'Chuantong Zhongguo yijie dui chengzhang yu fayu xianxiang de taolun' 傳統中國醫界對成長發育現象的討論 (Debates about growth and development in traditional Chinese medicine), *Guoli Taiwan shifan daxue lishi xuebao*, no. 20 (July 1992), pp. 27–40.

——, 'More or less: Cultural and medical factors behind marital fertility in late imperial China', paper presented at the IUSSP/IRCJS Workshop, Kyoto, 17–22 Oct. 1994.

——, 'Sons and mothers: Demographic realities and the Chinese culture of *hsiao*', paper presented at the Annual Meeting of the Association of Asian Studies, Hawaii, 11–14 April 1996.

——, *Youyou. Chuantong Zhongguo de qiangbao zhi dao* 幼幼：傳統中國 的襁褓之道 (The care of infants in traditional China), Taibei: Lianjing chuban shiye gongsi, 1995.

——, 'Zhongguo jinshi de xinsheng'er zhaohu' 中國近世的新生兒照 護 (Care for neonates in early modern China), *Zhongguo jinshi shehui wenhua shilun wenji* (Papers on society and culture in early modern China), Taibei: Academia Sinica, 1992, pp. 387–428.

——, 'Zhongguo jinshi shiren bixia de ertong jiankang wenti' 中國近世 士人筆下的兒童健康問題 (Problems of child health in the writings of the educated élite in early modern China), *Zhongyang yanjiuyuan jindaishi yanjiusuo jikan*, 23, no. 2 (June 1994), pp. 1–29.

Hsu, Francis L.K., *Under the ancestors' shadow: Chinese culture and personality*, London: Routledge and Kegan Paul, 1949.

Hutchinson, John, *The dynamics of cultural nationalism*, London: Geo. Allen and Unwin, 1987.

Huet, Marie-Hélène, *Monstrous imagination*, Cambridge, MA: Harvard University Press, 1993.

Hull, Terence H., *Recent population policy in China*, Australian International Development Assistance Bureau, Sector Report, no. 4, 1991.

Human Rights Watch, *Death by default: A policy of fatal neglect in China's state orphanages*, Human Rights Watch Report, January 1996.

Impey, Oliver and Arthur MacGregor, *The origins of museums: The cabinet of curiosities in sixteenth to seventeenth century Europe*, Oxford: Clarendon Press, 1985.

Jacquart, Denise and Claude Thomasset, *Sexuality and medicine in the Middle Ages*, Cambridge: Polity, 1988.

Jeambrun, Pascale, 'Regards de lune. Albinisme oculocutané', *Ethnologie Française*, 24, no. 1 (Jan.–March 1994), pp. 25–35.

Jia Zhizhong 賈治中 and Yang Yanfei 楊燕飛, 'Dashengbian ji qi zuozhe kao' 達生編及其作者考 (An inquiry into the *Dashengbian* and its author), *Zhonghua yishi zazhi*, 1994, 24, no. 3, pp. 183–5.

Johnson, Kay, 'Chinese orphanages: Saving China's abandoned girls', *Australian Journal of Chinese Studies*, no. 30 (July 1993), pp. 61–87.

Johnson, Linda Cooke (ed.), *Cities of Jiangnan in late imperial China*, Albany: State University of New York Press, 1993.

Jones, Steve, *In the blood: God, genes and destiny*, London: HarperCollins, 1996.

Jones-Davies, M.T. (ed.), *Monstres et prodiges au temps de la Renaissance*, Paris: Touzot, 1980.

Jordanova, Ludmilla (ed.), *Languages of nature: Critical essays on science and literature*, London: Free Association Books, 1986.

Kämpf, Klaus, *Teratologie als Vorstufe einer Entwicklungsgeschichte. A.W. Otto (1786–1845) und sein "Museum Monstrorum"*, Breslau 1841, Feuchtwangen: Kohlhauer, 1987.

Kane, Penny, *China and the one-child family*, New York: M. Russell, 1984.

Kaye, Lincoln, 'Quality control: Eugenics bill defended against Western critics', *Far Eastern Economic Review*, 13 January 1994, p. 22.

Keller, Evelyn Fox, *Refiguring life: Metaphors of twentieth-century biology*, New York: Columbia University Press, 1995.

Kevles, D.J., *In the name of eugenics: Genetics and the use of human heredity*, New York: Alfred Knopf, 1985.

King, Ambrose Y.C., 'The individual and group in Confucianism' in Donald J. Munro, *Individualism and holism: Studies in Confucian and Taoist values*, Ann Arbor: Center for Chinese Studies, 1985, pp. 57–70.

Ko, Dorothy, *Teachers of the inner chambers: Women and culture in seventeenth-century China*, Stanford University Press, 1994.

Kong Shuzhen 孔淑真, 'Songdai fuchan kexue' 宋代婦產科學 (Medicine for childbirth and women in the Song dynasty), *Zhonghua yishi zazhi*, 1994, no. 3, pp. 183–5.

Krauss, Richard Curt, 'Class conflict and the vocabulary of social analysis', *China Quarterly*, 69 (March 1977), pp. 54–74.

Kristof, Nicholas D., 'Parts of China forcibly sterilizing the retarded who wish to marry', *New York Times*, 15 August 1991, p. 1.

Larson, Edward J., *Sex, race, and science: Eugenics in the Deep South*, Baltimore: Johns Hopkins University Press, 1996.

Laufer, Berthold, 'Sex transformation and hermaphrodites in China', *American Journal of Physical Anthropology*, 3, no. 2 (1920), reprinted in *Kleinere Schriften von Berthold Laufer*, Wiesbaden: Franz Steiner Verlag, 1979, part 2, pp. 1306–9.

Laqueur, Thomas W., *Making sex: Body and gender from the Greeks to Freud*, Cambridge, MA: Harvard University Press, 1990.

Le Minor, Jean-Marie, 'Les "Fasciculi Admirandorum Naturae" (1679–83) du strasbourgeois F.M. Schmuck et la tératologie', *Histoire des Sciences Médicales*, 27 (1993), pp. 311–20.

Lee, James and Robert Eng, 'Population and family history in eighteenth-century Manchuria: Preliminary results from Daoyi, 1774–1798', *Ch'ing-shih wen-t'i*, 5, no. 1 (June 1984), pp. 1–55.

Lee, James Z. and Cameron D. Campbell, *Fate and fortune in rural China: Social organization and popular behaviour in Liaoning, 1774–1873*, Cambridge University Press, 1997.

Leung, Angela K. C., 'Organized medicine in Ming-Qing China: State and private medical institutions in the Lower Yangzi region', *Late Imperial China*, 8, no. 1 (June 1987), pp. 134–66.

Leung, Angela K. C. 梁其姿, *Shishan yu jiaohua: Ming Qing de cishan zuzhi* 施善與教化：明清的慈善組織 (Charity and civilisation: Charitable organisations in the Ming and the Qing), Taibei: Lianjing chuban shiye gongsi, 1997.

Levine, Philippa, *The amateur and the professional: Antiquarians, historians and archaeologists in Victorian England, 1838–1886*, Cambridge University Press, 1986.

Li Chunsheng 李春生, 'Ming Qing zhi jiefang qian yangsheng fazhan shi gai' 明清至解放前養生發展史概 (An overview of the history of the unfolding of *yangsheng* from the Ming and the Qing to liberation), *Zhonghua yishi zazhi*, 1989, 19, no. 2, pp. 71–5.

Li Jen-der 李真德, 'Han Tang zhijian qiuzi yifang shitan: jianlun fuke lanshang yu xingbie lunshu' 漢唐之間求子醫方試探：兼論婦科濫觴與性別論述 (Reproductive medicine in late antiquity and early medieval China: Gender discourse and the birth of gynecology), *Zhongyang yanjiuyuan lishi yuyan yanjiu jikan*, 68, no. 2 (July 1997), pp. 283–367.

Li Jinyuan 李今垣, 'Chen Shiduo ji qi zhuzuo' 陳士鐸及其著作 (Chen Shiduo and his work), *Zhonghua yishi zazhi*, 1988, 18, no. 1, pp. 20–4.

Liao Yuqun 廖育群, 'Xiaoshan zhulinsi nüke kaolüe' 蕭山竹林寺女科考略 (Investigation of the work on medicine for women of the Temple of the Bamboo Grove monastery in Xiaoshan), *Zhonghua yishi zazhi*, 1986, 16, no. 3, pp. 159–61.

Liu, James T.C., *China turning inwards: Intellectual-political changes in the early twelfth century*, Cambridge, MA: Harvard University Press, 1988.

Ma Dazheng 馬大正, *Zhongguo fuchanke fazhan shi* 中國婦產科發展史 (History of medicine for women and childbirth in China), Taiyuan: Shanxi kexue jiaoyu chubanshe, 1991.

Mannix, Daniel P., *Freaks: We who are not as others. With rare and amazing photos from the author's personal scrapbook*, San Francisco: Research Publications, 1990.

Marx, Jacques, 'Descriptions géographiques et mythiques au XVIIe siècle', *Revue Roumaine d'Histoire*, 22, no. 4 (1983), pp. 357–69.

McDermott, Joseph P., 'The Chinese domestic bursar', *Ajia bunka kenkyu*, no. 2 (Nov. 1990), pp. 284–67.

Michler, Andrea Gloria, 'Ambiguità e transmutazione. Discussioni mediche e giuridiche in epoca moderna (secoli XVII e XVIII)', *Memoria i Revista di Storia delle Donne*, no. 24 (1988), pp. 43–60.

'"More babies move" for China's well-educated', *Straits Times*, 29 Aug. 1996.

Moscucci, Ornella, 'Hermaphroditism and sex difference: The construction of gender in Victorian England' in Marina Benjamin (ed.), *Science and sensibility: Gender and scientific enquiry, 1780–1945*, London: Blackwell, 1991, pp. 174–99.

Niquet, Valérie, 'The family on the chessboard of power politics', *China News Analysis*, no. 1561, 1 June 1996, pp. 1–10.

Nisot, M.T., *La question eugénique dans les divers pays*, Brussels: Falk, 1927–9.

Noordman, Jan, *Om de kwaliteit van het nageslacht. Eugenetika in Nederland, 1900–1950*, Nijmegen: SUN, 1989.

Nye, Robert, 'The rise and fall of the eugenics empire: Recent perspectives on the impact of bio-medical thought in modern society', *Historical Journal*, 36, no. 3 (1993), pp. 687–700.

Park, K. and L.J. Daston, 'Unnatural conceptions: The study of monsters in sixteenth- and seventeenth-century France and England', *Past and Present*, no. 92 (August 1981), pp. 20–54.

Pauly, P.J., 'Review article: The eugenics industry – Growth or restructuring?', *Journal of the History of Biology*, 26, no. 1 (spring 1993), pp. 131–45.

Pearson, Veronica, 'Health and responsibility: But whose?' in Linda Wong and Steward MacPherson (eds), *Social change and social policy in China*, Aldershot: Avebury, 1995, pp. 88–112.

——, *Mental health care in China: State policies, professional services and family responsibilities*, London: Gaskell, 1995.

——, 'Population policy and eugenics in China', *British Journal of Psychiatry*, 167 (1995), pp. 1–4.

Peng Xizhe, *Demographic transition in China: Fertility trends since the 1950s*, Oxford: Clarendon Press, 1991.

Pernick, Martin S., *The black stork: Eugenics and the death of 'defective' babies in American medicine and motion pictures since 1915*, Oxford University Press, 1996.

Pomata, Gianna, 'Uomini mestruanti: Somiglianza e differenza fra i sessi in età moderna', *Quaderni Storici*, no. 1 (1992), pp. 51–103.

Porter, Roy, 'Gentlemen and geology: The emergence of a scientific career, 1660–1920', *Historical Journal*, no. 21 (1978), pp. 809–36.

——, 'Love, sex, and madness in eighteenth-century England', *Social Research*, no. 53 (1986), pp. 211–42.

——, *Mind-forg'd manacles: A history of madness in England from the Restoration to the Regency*, London: Penguin Books, 1990.

Pouchelle, Marie-Christine, *The body and surgery in the Middle Ages*, New Brunswick, NJ: Rutgers University Press, 1990.

Praag, P. van, *Het bevolkingsvraagstuk in Nederland. Ontwikkeling van standpunten en opvattingen (1918–1940)*, Deventer: Van Loghum Slaterus, 1976.

Preiswerk, Frank, 'Auguste Forel (1848–1931). Un projet de régénération sociale, morale et raciale', *Annuelles. Revue d'Histoire Contemporaine*, 2 (1991), pp. 25–50.

Proctor, Robert N., *Racial hygiene: Medicine under the Nazis*, Cambridge, MA: Harvard University Press, 1988.

Rawski, Evelyn S., 'Economic and social foundations of late imperial culture' in David Johnson, Andrew J. Nathan and Evelyn S. Rawski (eds), *Popular culture in late imperial China*, Berkeley: University of California Press, 1985, pp. 3–33.

——, *Education and popular literacy in Ch'ing China*, Ann Arbor: University of Michigan Press, 1979.

Richards, Evelleen, 'A political anatomy of monsters, hopeful or otherwise: Teratogeny, transcendentalism, and evolutionary theorizing', *Isis*, 85 (1994), pp. 377–411.

Russett, Cynthia E., *Sexual science: The Victorian construction of womanhood*, Cambridge, MA: Harvard University Press, 1989.

Schmuhl, Hans-Walter, *Rassenhygiene, Nationalsozialismus, Euthanasie*, Göttingen: Vandenhoeck und Ruprecht, 1987.

Schneider, Laurence A., 'Genetics in Republican China' in J.Z. Bowers, J.W. Hess and N. Sivin (eds), *Science and medicine in twentieth-century China: Research and education*, Ann Arbor: Center for Chinese Studies, 1988, pp. 3–30.

——, 'Learning from Russia: Lysenkoism and the fate of genetics in China, 1950–1986' in Merle Goldman and Denis F. Simon (eds), *Science and technology in post-Mao China*, Cambridge, MA: Harvard University Press, 1989, pp. 45–65.

——, *Lysenkoism in China: Proceedings of the 1956 Qingdao Genetics Symposium*, Armonk, NY: M.E. Sharpe, 1986.

Schneider, William H., *Quality and quantity: The quest for biological regeneration in twentieth-century France*, Cambridge University Press, 1990.

Shapiro, Hugh L., 'The view from a Chinese asylum: Defining madness in 1930s Peking', unpublished Ph.D. diss., Harvard University, 1995.

Sheng Weizhong 盛維忠, '*Waike lili ji Wang Ji de waike xueshu sixiang*', 外科理例及汪機的外科學術思想 (The *Principles of Surgery* of Wang Ji and his knowledge of surgery), *Zhonghua yishi zazhi*, 1985, 15, no. 1, pp. 48–53.

Sonderegger, Albert, *Missgeburten und Wundergestalten in Einblattdrucken und Handzeichnungen des 16. Jahrhunderts*, Zürich: Füssli, 1927.

Song Chien, *Population control in China: Theory and applications*, New York: Praeger, 1985.

Spence, Jonathan D., 'Collapse of a purist' in *Chinese roundabout: Essays in history and culture*, New York: W.W. Norton, 1992, pp. 124–31.

Spufford, Margaret, *Small books and pleasant histories: Popular fiction and its readership in seventeenth-century England*, Cambridge University Press, 1989.

Stepan, Nancy L., *'The hour of eugenics': Race, gender, and nation in Latin America*, Ithaca: Cornell University Press, 1991.

——, 'Eugenics in Brazil, 1917–1940' in Mark B. Adams (ed.), *The well-born science: Eugenics in Germany, France, Brazil and Russia*, Oxford University Press, 1990, pp. 110–216.

Strathern, Marilyn, *Reproducing the future: Anthropology, kinship and the new reproductive technologies*, Manchester University Press, 1992.

Taguieff, Pierre-André, 'Eugénisme ou décadence? L'exception française', *Ethnologie Française*, 24, no. 1 (Jan.–March 1994), pp. 81–103.

Thurston, Anne F., 'In a Chinese orphanage', *The Atlantic Monthly*, 277, no. 4 (April 1996), pp. 28–41.

Tien, Yuan H., 'China's population planning after Tiananmen', *Population Today*, 18, no. 9 (1990), pp. 6–8.

Todd, Dennis, *Imagining monsters: Miscreations of the self in eighteenth-century England*, University of Chicago Press, 1995.

Tong Guangdong 童光東, Wang Letao 王樂匋 and Xu Yecheng 許業誠, 'Ming Qing shiqi Hui ban yiji ji qi yishi zuoyong' 明清時期徽版醫籍及其醫史作用 (Medical publications printed in Anhui during the Ming and the Qing and their function in medical history), *Zhonghua yishi zazhi*, 1989, 19, no. 4, pp. 242–46.

Tong Guangdong 童光東 and Liu Huiling 劉惠玲, 'Ming Qing shiqi Xin'an yaodian ji qi yiyaoxue zuoyong' 明清時期新安藥店及其醫藥學作用 (Xin'an dispensaries and their role in the Ming and Qing), *Zhonghua yishi zazhi*, 1995, 25, no. 1, pp. 30–4.

Tort, Patrick, *L'ordre et les monstres. Le débat sur l'origine des déviations anatomiques au XVIIIe siècle*, Paris: Le Sycomore, 1980.

Tsay, Queenie, 'Chinese superstitions relating to child-birth', *China Medical Journal*, 32, no. 5 (Sept. 1918), p. 533.

Tyler, Patrick E., 'Lacking iodine in their diets, millions in China are retarded', *New York Times*, 4 June 1996, p. A1.

Unschuld, Paul U., 'Epistemological issues and changing legitimation: Traditional Chinese medicine in the twentieth century' in Charles Leslie and Allan Young (eds), *Paths to Asian medical knowledge*, Berkeley: University of California Press, 1992, pp. 44–61.

——, *Medicine in China: A history of ideas*, Berkeley: University of California Press, 1985.

Vigarello, Georges, *Le corps redressé. Histoire d'un pouvoir pédagogique*, Paris: Delarge, 1978.

——, 'The upward training of the body from the age of chivalry to courtly civility' in Michel Feher with Ramona Naddaff and Nadia Tazi (eds), *Fragments for a history of the human body*, New York: Zone Books, 1989, vol. 2, pp. 148–99.

von Senger, Harro, 'Erbgesundheitslehre in der Volksrepublik China' in Jarmila Bedbaríková and Frank C. Chapmann (eds), *Festschrift für Jan Stepán*, Zürich: Schulthess Polygraphischer Verlag, 1994, pp. 219–32.

Walton, M.T., R.M. Fineman and P.J. Walton, 'Of monsters and prodigies: The interpretation of birth defects in the sixteenth century', *American Journal of Medical Genetics*, 47, no. 1 (Aug. 1993), pp. 7–13.

Weindling, Paul J., *Health, race and German politics between national unification and Nazism, 1870–1945*, Cambridge University Press, 1989.

Weingart, Peter, Jörgen Kroll and Kurt Bayertz, *Rasse, Blut und Gene. Geschichte der Eugenik und Rassenhygiene in Deutschland*, Frankfurt am Main: Suhrkamp, 1988.

White, Gordon, *The politics of class and class origin: The case of the Cultural Revolution*, Canberra: Australian National University, 1976.

Whyte, Martin King, 'Urban life in the People's Republic' in Roderick MacFarquhar and John K. Fairbank (eds), *The Cambridge history of China*, Vol. 15: *The People's Republic, part 2: Revolutions within the Chinese revolution, 1966–1982*, Cambridge University Press, 1991, pp. 682–742.

Widmer, Ellen, 'The Huanduzhai of Hangzhou and Suzhou: A study in seventeenth-century publishing', *Harvard Journal of Asiatic Studies*, 56, no. 1 (1996), pp. 77–122.

Wile, Douglas, *Art of the bedchamber: The Chinese sexual yoga classics including women's solo meditation texts*, Albany: State University of New York Press, 1992.

Wilson, Dudley, *Signs and portents: Monstrous births from the Middle Ages to the Enlightenment*, London: Routledge, 1993.

Wilson, Philip K., '"Out of sight, out of mind?": The Daniel Turner-James Blondel dispute over the power of the maternal imagination', *Annals of Science*, no. 49 (1992), pp. 159–97.

Wolff, Etienne, *La science des monstres*, Paris: Gallimard, 1948.

Wu Yi-Li, 'Transmitted secrets: The doctors of the lower Yangzi region and "medicine for women" in late imperial China', unpublished Ph.D. diss., Yale University, 1998.

Xu Ji'ou 徐寄鷗, 'Shen Jin'ao xiansheng zhuanlüe' 沈金鰲先生傳略 (A brief biography of Shen Jin'ao), *Jiangsu zhongyi*, 34 (1963), p. 3.

Xue Qinglu (ed.) 薛清录, *Quanguo zhongyi tushu lianhe mulu* 全國中醫

圖書聯合目录 (Combined catalogue of publications in Chinese medicine), Beijing: Zhongyi guji chubanshe, 1991.

Yip Ka-che, *Health and national reconstruction in nationalist China: The development of modern health services, 1928–1937*, Ann Arbor: Association for Asian Studies, 1995.

Zanca, Attilio, 'In tema di hypertrichosis universalis congenita: Contributo storico-medico', *Physis*, 25, no. 1 (1983), pp. 41–66.

Zapperi, Roberto, 'Arrigo le velu, Pietro le fou, Amon le nain et autres bêtes: Autour d'un tableau d'Agostino Carrache', *Annales. Économies, Sociétés, Civilisations*, 40, no. 2 (1987), pp. 307–27.

Zeitlin, Judith, *Historian of the strange: Pu Songling and his Chinese classical tale*, Stanford University Press, 1993.

Zhou Lenian 周樂年 and Jiang Weizhou 姜衛周, *Zhongyi youshengxue* 中醫優生學 (Eugenics in traditional Chinese medicine), Beijing: Kexue jishu wenxian chubanshe, 1991.

Zhou Yimou 周一謀, *Zhongguo gudai fangshi yangshengxue* 中國古代房事養生學 (The science of sex in ancient China), Beijing: Zhongwai wenhua chubanshe, 1989.

——, *Mawangdui Hanmu chutu: Fangzhong yangsheng* 馬王堆漢墓出土：房中養生 (The Mawangdui excavations from Han tombs: The art of the bedchamber and the nourishment of life), Hong Kong: Haifeng chubanshe, 1990.

CHARACTER LIST

baichi 白癡
Beiji qianjin yaofang 備急千金
　要方
biji 筆記
bushen 補腎
buxue 補血

Cai Yuanpei 蔡元培
Cao Guanlai 曹觀來
chanke 產科
Chen Changheng 陳長衡
Chen Da 陳達
chengui louxi 陳規陋習
Chen Jianshan 陳兼善
Chen Lifu 陳立夫
Chen Minzhang 陳敏章
Chen Muhua 陳慕華
Chen Shiduo 陳士鐸
Chen Tianbiao 陳天表
Chen Yucang 陳雨蒼
Chen Zhen 陳楨
chongji 衝擊
chiyu 癡愚
chumu jingxin 觸目驚心
chunfangyao 春方藥
cipin 次品
Cong Li 從利
cun tianli mie renyu 存天理滅
　人慾

Dashengbian 達生編
Dasheng yaozhi 大生要旨
daiben 呆笨
Dai Sigong 戴思恭
daixie wuzhi 代謝物質
Dai Zhi 戴幟
daizi 呆子
dan 淡
Danxi 丹溪
denggao 登高
dineng 低能
dianxian 癲癇
Ding Shu'an 丁淑安

Dongyuan 東垣
duo dianzi taijiao yi 多電子胎
　教儀
duotaiyao 墮胎藥

erke 兒科

faxian 發現
fanben yichuan 返本遺傳
fanying 反應
Fang Lizhi 方勵之
fangzhong 房中
fei (fat) 肥
fei (lungs) 肺
feipin 非品
fei yichuan de xiantian jibing
　非遺傳的先天疾病
feiyong 肺癰
fenlei xiedou 分類械鬥
fengjian 封建
fuke 婦科
Fu Shan 傅山

gan 肝
ganshou muqi 感受母氣
Gao Jinsheng 高錦聲
Gao Xisheng 高希聖
Gong Zizhen 龔自珍
Gu Donggao 顧棟高
guaitai 怪胎
guiguai xingxiang 鬼怪形象
guisui 鬼祟
guitai 鬼胎
guixiong 鬼胸
Gui Youguang 歸有光
Gui Zhiliang 桂質良
guojia 國家
guomin 國民

hongdong quanshi 轟動全市
Hong Liangji 洪亮吉
Hu Buchan 胡步蟾
huajing 滑精

219

huanjing 還精
huangbo 黃柏
huangdi zisun 黃帝子孫
Huang Yuanyu 黃元御
huangzhong 黃種

jiben yinsu 基本因素
jitaixue 畸胎學
jixing'er 畸形兒
jixing guaizhuang 畸形怪狀
jixiong 雞胸
jiyin 基因
jiyinku 基因庫
Jiating jianghua 家庭講話
jiaxing ban yinyang 假性半陰陽
jiazuxing xiaotou 家族性小頭
jiankang youyi 健康有益
jieji 階級
jiejue 解決
jieyu 節慾
jinhua 進化
jing (quiescence) 靜
jing 精
jingshenbing 精神病
jingshen fayu buliang 精神發育
   不良
junhuo 君火

kangyang 亢陽
Kang Youwei 康有為
Ke Jia 柯炘
kexue 科學
kexue rendaozhuyi 科學人道
   主義
kongzhi 控制
ku 苦
kuangdian 狂癲
laozhai 癆瘵
leng 冷
Li Chan 李梴

Li Gao 李杲
Liji 禮記

Li Mingzhi 李明之
Li Peng 李鵬
Li Shizhen 李時珍
Li Xiaowei 李小衛
Li Yurong 李玉蓉
liyue 禮樂
lianghan 涼寒
Liang Qichao 梁啟超
Lienüzhuan 列女傳
liesheng 劣生
liesheng youbai 劣勝優敗
ling suzhi 零素質
Liu Piji 劉丕基
luanjing 亂精
luanxing 亂性
luohou 落後

maoren 毛人
meili fengguang 美麗風光
mengyi 夢遺
mixin 迷心
miezhong 滅種
miezu 滅族
minzu 民族
mingmen 命門
Mu Guangzong 穆光宗

nangyong 囊癰
ni taotai 逆淘汰
niaoxue 尿血
Niu Manjiang 牛滿江
nuqi 怒氣

Pan Gongzhan 潘公展
Pan Guangdan 潘光旦
Peng Peiyun 彭珮雲
pi 脾
pianshi 偏食
pingxin dingqi 平心定氣
pingxue 平血

qi 氣
qiguan xingchengzhi 器官形成質

Qi Sihe 齊思和
qiang 強
Qian Xinzhong 錢信忠
qiaomangyan 雀盲眼
Qin Huitian 秦蕙田
qingdu zhiruo 輕度智弱
qingxin guayu 清心寡慾
Qiu Renzong 邱仁宗
qiusi 求嗣

ranseti 染色體
re 熱
reyao 熱藥
renkou 人口
renzhong 人種
renzhong gailiang 人種改良
Ru Song 如松
ruo 弱

Sancai tuhua 三才圖劃
Santai wanyong zhengzong 三台
  萬用正宗
sanyou buwan 三友補丸
seqing zhongshu 色情中樞
shaixuan 篩選
shangzhi 上智
Shao Lizi 邵力子
shehui wenti 社會問題
shen 腎
Shen Jin'ao 沈金鰲
shenjing shuairuo 神精衰弱
shenshe chidai 伸舌癡呆
shengdihuang 生地黃
shengjiang 生姜
shengjiang 生僵
shengwuzhong 生物鍾
Shi Lu 史廬
shou 瘦
shuzhongxue 淑種學
si 思
simu 思慕
suzao chengxing 塑造成形
suan 酸

sui mu tingwen 隨母聽聞
Sun Benwen 孫本文
Sun Simo 孫思邈

taijiao 胎教
taijiao huatong 胎教話筒
taijiaoyuan 胎教院
Tang Qianqing 唐千頃
Tu Xing 屠興
tuihua 退化
tuihua tubian 退化突變
waijie ciji 外界刺激
waixiang er neigan 外象而內感
Wan Quan 萬全
Wang Chengpin 王誠品
Wang Ji 汪機
Wang Kentang 王肯堂
Wang Lun 王綸
Wang Qishu 王其澍
Wang Ruizi 王瑞梓
Wang Shiduo 汪士鐸
Wang Shishan 汪石山
Wang Wei 王偉
Wang Yanchang 王燕昌
Wang Yang 汪洋
wei 胃
weishengsu 衛生素
Wei Zhixiu 魏之琇
wenbu 溫補
wenren 文人
wenti 問題
wuchi 五遲
Wu Min 吳旻
Wu Qian 吳謙
wuruan 五軟

xiayu 下愚
xian 鹹
xiangshu 相術
xiangfa 相法
xianghuo 相火
xin (acrid) 辛
xin (heart) 心

xinli weisheng 心理衛生
xinshang 欣賞
xing (shape) 形
xingti buquan 形體不全
xingti canji 形體殘疾
Xu Dachun 徐大椿
Xu Shilian 許仕廉
xuanyou qulie 選優祛劣
xue 血
Xue Banghua 薛邦華
Xue Ji 薛己

Yan Chunxi 閻純璽
Yan Fu 顏復
Yan Yuan 顏元
yangjing 養精
Yang Nairong 楊乃榮
yangqi 養氣
yangsheng 養生
yaoren 妖人
yichuanbing 遺傳病
yichuanxue 遺傳學
yijing 遺精
Yizong jinjian 醫宗金鑑
yinhuan 隱患
yinqi zaoxie 陰氣早瀉
yinxing jiyin 隱形基因
yinyangren 陰陽人
yinyu zhi guo 隱慾之過
yingyangsu 營養素
you guilü de shenghuo 有規律
    的生活
You Jiade 游嘉德
yousheng 優生
yousheng liebai 優勝劣敗
youshengxue 優生學
yousi 優死
You Yi 尤怡
Yu Chang 喻昌
yudong 慾動
yufang 預防
Yu Fengbin 俞鳳賓

Yu Jingrang 于景讓
Yu Zhenhuan 于震環
yuanhou zisun 猿猴子孫
Yuan Huarong 原華榮
yuanqi 元氣
yuanxian 猿線
Yue Fujia 岳甫嘉

zaisha xiongwu 宰殺凶惡
zaoxie 早瀉
Zhang Boxing 張伯行
Zhang Jiebin 張介賓
Zhang Jingsheng 張競生
Zhang Junjun 張君俊
Zhang Xueliang 張學良
Zhang Yaosun 張曜孫
Zhang Zuoren 張作人
Zhao Gongmin 趙功民
Zhao Xianke 趙獻可
zhesixue 哲嗣學
zhenxing ban yinyang 真性半
    陰陽
zhengchang de xingtai 正常的
    形態
zhili dixia 智力低下
zhineng di 智能低
zhong 種
zhongzi 種子
zhongzu 種族
Zhou Dunyi 周敦頤
Zhou Efen 周咢芬
Zhou Jianren 周建人
Zhou Xianzhi 周顯志
Zhou Xiaozheng 周孝正
Zhu Xi 朱洗
Zhu Xi 朱熹
Zhu Zhenheng 朱震亨
ziran 自然
ziyin 滋陰
ziyin wenbu 滋陰溫補
zu 族
Zuo Zongtang 左宗棠

INDEX

abortifacients, 28, 56, 59
adolescence, 131–2
age, 43, 131–2
agency, 69, 71; *see* causality,
   responsibility
albinism, 47, 90
alcohol, 34, 40, 45, 48, 100, 107,
   118, 130–1, 150
amenorrhea, 53, 56; *see also*
   menstruation
analogical thinking, 32, 45–8, 57,
   100–2, 132, 148
aphrodisiacs, 42–3

birth control, 109–10, 123; *see also*
   population policies
blood, 23, 33–43, 97; *see also*
   menstruation
bodily fluids, 17, 33, 76; *see also*
   menstruation, semen
body, 9, 33, 69, 135
Brazil, 4–5, 118
Britain, 3–5, 116, 130

Cai Yuanpei, 102–3, 113
Cao Guanlai, 99
Cao Tingdong, 107
castration, 107
causality, 10, 69, 125–7, 150, 151; *see*
   also agency, responsibility
Chen Changheng, 113
Chen Da, 110, 113
Chen Jianshan, 73, 110
Chen Lifu, 113
Chen Minzhang, 166
Chen Muhua, 162, 166
Chen Shiduo, 35, 52
Chen Tianbiao, 111
Chen Yucang, 85, 90
Chen Zhen, 73
Cheng-Zhu Confucianism, 17, 31–2,
   50

Chow Kai-wing, 31
class, 4, 108–10, 120–2, 133
climate, 45, 102, 126, 132–3; *see also*
   environment, pollution
cloning, *see* reproductive
   technologies
Confucianism, 103, 138; *see also*
   kaozhengxue, Cheng-Zhu
   Confucianism, Han Confucianism
Cong Li, 162
consanguinity, 154
contraception, 28; *see also* birth
   control
correlative thinking, 40, 44, 47; *see*
   also analogical thinking,
   cosmology, holism, medicine of
   systematic correspondence
cosmology, 17, 32, 36, 44, 45, 65,
   132
criminality, 99, 107, 110, 112
criminology, 4
Cultural Revolution, 121

Dai Sigong, 23
Dai Zhi, 145
Danxi, 23–6
demonology, 14, 56
demographic change, 26
Denmark, 3, 115
Deng Xiaoping, 122
diet, 40–1, 45, 47–8, 101–2
Ding Shu'an, 91
disease, 10, 37, 125–6, 128–30
Dongyuan, 24–6, 34, 54

economic change, 21, 64, 124
education, 5, 50, 103–5; *see also*
   taijiao
embryology, 75–6, 91–3
emotions, 40, 45, 48–50, 52–4,
   97–100, 146–8

223